Assessing Organizational Readiness for Capitation

Jennings Ryan & Kolb, Inc.

Edited by
Deborah S. Kolb, PhD

AHA books are published by American Hospital Publishing, Inc., an American Hospital Association company

This publication is designed to provide accurate and authoritative information in regard to the subject matter covered. It is sold with the understanding that neither the authors nor the publisher is engaged in rendering legal, accounting, or other professional service. If legal advice or other expert assistance is required, the services of a competent professional person should be sought.

The views expressed in this publication are strictly those of the authors and do not necessarily represent official positions of the American Hospital Association.

Library of Congress Cataloging-in-Publication Data

Assessing organizational readiness for capitation / edited by Deborah
    S. Kolb.
        p.   cm.
    Includes bibliographical references.
    ISBN 1-55648-154-3
    1. Hospitals—Business management.   2. Hospital—Finance.
3. Insurance, Health.   I. Kolb, Deborah S.
    [DNLM: 1. Economics, Hospital—organization & administration.
    2. Capitation Fee.   3. Prepaid Health Plans—organization &
administration.   4. Organizational Innovation.   WX 157 A846 1995]
    RA971.3.A766   1995
    362.1'1'0681—dc20
    DNLM/DLC
    for Library of Congress   96-4580
                                                                                CIP

Catalog no. 131002

Printed in the USA

ᴀʜᴀ is a service mark of the American Hospital Association used under license by American Hospital Publishing, Inc.

Text set in Times

3M—3/96—0434

Richard Hill, Senior Editor
Lee Benaka, Editor
Peggy DuMais, Assistant Manager, Production
Marcia Bottoms, Books Division Director

This work is dedicated to our leader,

Marian C. Jennings.

Assessing Organizational Readiness for Capitation

Most health care organizations recognize the need to understand capitation and prepare for its arrival in their markets. Preparing for capitation, however, is not simple; significant organizational trauma, not to mention expense and effort, is involved.

Members of health care organizations have been inundated with information about capitation, and they may feel overwhelmed by the prospect of preparing for capitation. Furthermore, sometimes individual members of health care organizations focus on the aspects of capitation that are most accessible or understandable to them. For example, a member of the finance department who is familiar with management information systems may focus on the need for better cost accounting data. A medical director may be inclined to emphasize the need for practice protocols or guidelines. The goal of this book is to provide an overview of capitation pertinent to the organization as a whole, so that the organization's leaders can establish priorities and balance the needs of all constituencies.

Through our consulting work we have seen organizations thrive under capitation, but we also have seen organizations suffer. Such experiences led us to ask ourselves the question: Which attributes are associated with the health care organizations that thrive? Through the distillation of anecdotal evidence from our experiences with capitation, we concluded that two dimensions are crucial to capitation readiness: structural readiness and information systems readiness. (A third key dimension that we have not been able to define or quantify satisfactorily is leadership readiness.)

In order to thrive under capitation, organizations must have information systems that facilitate the management of risk and the monitoring of costs of care. But sophisticated information systems alone will not ensure success. Organizations also need structures in place to deal with the new demands, behaviors, and conflicts inherent in capitation, such as:

- The need for more primary care providers and "gatekeepers"
- The need to develop panels of providers for risk contracts
- The need to respond to the market quickly
- The need to mediate the potentially conflicting interests of hospital, physicians, and patients

This book presents an organizational readiness survey instrument that Jennings Ryan & Kolb has used to help clients identify their critical needs as they prepare for capitation. Among other things, this tool can be used to:

- Facilitate discussion of capitation at planning retreats involving hospital managers, board members, and physicians. Retreat members can break into small groups that include members of each constituency, fill out the survey instrument, and then compare their responses with others to identify areas of agreement or disagreement.
- Help set priorities for the most important steps that need to be taken near term, then longer term, in order to move the organization toward readiness for capitation.

- Identify areas of agreement and/or disagreement among management team members concerning the organization's readiness for capitation.
- Educate department managers and other constituencies about organizational changes associated with capitation.
- Measure progress toward capitation readiness from year to year.

This book follows the format of the organizational readiness tool itself: the first half covers the 10 components of structural readiness, and the second half discusses the 10 components of information readiness. The following section explains how the survey instrument is structured.

Using the Self-Assessment Tool

The organizational readiness self-assessment tool is shown on the next two pages. There are two survey dimensions to the tool: structural readiness for capitation and information readiness for capitation. Both survey dimensions consist of a series of 10 statements, each followed by a scoring grid. Survey participants should read each statement and decide whether it describes their present organization. Then participants should circle their scoring selection for each item and total the number of points circled. Scores in the column labeled "In Progress/ Needs Improvement" should be circled if the participant believes that significant effort has been expended to implement the feature being described but implementation has not yet been completed or fully succeeded. The far right-hand column lists the page in this book on which each criterion is discussed.

There is no magic in the scores assigned to each survey item. The scores reflect our judgment of the importance of these features to the success of integrated systems with which we are familiar. In some cases we stressed the importance of a feature by assigning a zero to features that are in progress or need improvement.

Organizational Readiness Self-Assessment Tool: Structural Readiness for Capitation

Structural Readiness	No	In Progress/ Needs Improvement	Yes	Discussed on Page
1. All major constituencies, including physicians, senior management, department directors, and board members, have a basic understanding of capitation.	0	0	1	10
2. Top management emphasizes and rewards innovation and prudent risk taking.	0	0	1	14
3. Hospital/system has ownership of or tight contractual relationships with facilities and services to provide a full continuum of care (accounts for at least 90 percent of the non-professional costs of health care).	0	1	3	16
4. Hospital/system has a strong, tightly aligned, and geographically dispersed primary care base.	0	1	2	21
5. Physicians are actively involved in using case mix, cost, and quality information to improve hospital service delivery.	0	1	2	26
6. Physicians and management work well together, and trust levels are high.	0	0	1	28
7. Excellent concurrent review and utilization review functions are in place.	0	1	2	31
8. Interdepartmental cooperation is very good. The hospital uses a "team" approach and has moved away from a traditional (hierarchical) organization.	0	1	2	34
9. Hospital/system has the financial resources to absorb any start-up "losses" due to innovative contractual arrangements.	0	1	3	37
10. The hospital and affiliated physicians have formed a contracting organization (for example, a PHO) that is legally and organizationally empowered to enter into risk contracts for all members.	0	1	3	39

Total Structural Readiness = _____

Organizational Readiness Self-Assessment Tool: Information Readiness for Capitation

Information Readiness	No	In Progress/ Needs Improvement	Yes	Discussed on Page
1. Physicians can schedule patients and obtain results reporting directly via office computers.	0	1	2	43
2. Hospital/system is actively developing a database of current experience that links hospital, physician, and other affiliated providers' data to track services rendered to a patient throughout an "episode of care."	0	1	2	45
3. A computerized quality/outcome measurement system is in place.	0	1	2	48
4. Clinical protocols or norms are established and monitored for selected procedures/cases.	0	1	2	51
5. Employer group and specific insurance plan are coded and accessible for all patients.	0	0	1	56
6. Information system provides up-to-date tracking of which managed care plans physicians participate in.	0	1	2	58
7. A cost accounting system provides accurate fixed, variable, and total costs at a procedure level, which then can be aggregated to a patient case.	0	1	3	62
8. A case mix system provides volumes, payment amounts, and costs (if available) by procedure, DRG, physician, payer, day of stay, and so forth.	0	1	2	67
9. Flexible reporting is available (for example, special reports can be produced easily).	0	1	2	73
10. Hospital/system has a market database that provides profiles of area managed care plans, analyses of service area population and managed care enrollment, and competitor information.	0	1	2	75

Total Information Readiness = _____

The following organizational matrix should be used by participants to plot their response scores. The matrix allows participants to easily visualize the strengths and weaknesses of their organization. For example, members of one hospital completed the readiness assessment and scored 15 points for information readiness but only 7 for structural readiness. The hospital's score placed it in the lower right-hand quadrant labeled "Strengthen Organization," which suggested that the hospital's improvement efforts needed to focus primarily on structural issues in the near term.

Scoring Matrix for Self-Assessment Tool

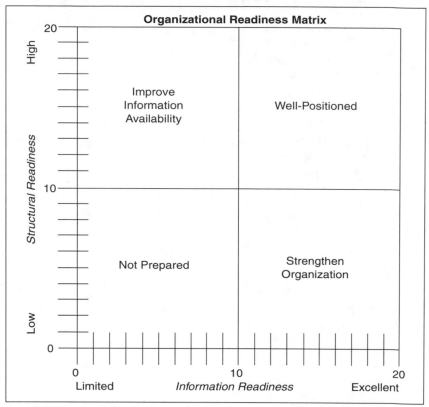

Copyright Jennings Ryan & Kolb, Inc. Reproduction in any form is forbidden without the express permission of copyright holder.

Using the Self-Assessment Tool

Assessing Structural Readiness

The following sections discuss the 10 structural readiness criteria. The importance of each criterion is explained, and then some or all of the following questions are answered for each:

- What is needed to answer yes?
- What about partial credit?
- Where are most organizations today?

Criterion 1

Structural Readiness	No	In Progress/ Needs Improvement	Yes
1. All major constituencies, including physicians, senior management, department directors, and board members, have a basic understanding of capitation.	0	0	1

Why Is an Understanding of Capitation Important for All Constituencies?

Under the traditional fee-for-service reimbursement structure, providers' revenues are directly proportional to the volume of health care services provided. The fee-for-service reimbursement model is similar to that found in most modern industries: once break-even volume is reached, profitability increases as volume increases. Therefore, under fee-for-service reimbursement, hospitals and physicians are motivated to generate more profits by providing more services to patients. Figure 1 shows the economics of fee-for-service health care.

The economics of capitated health care are the opposite of fee-for-service economics. Under capitation, provider revenues equal a fixed per-member, per-month fee times the number of enrolled lives under contract. Thus, for a given number of enrollees, provider revenues are fixed regardless of the volume or cost of health care the enrollees receive. Unlike the fee-for-service model, where profitability increases as volume increases, provider profitability decreases under capitation as more and more health care is provided. Figure 2 shows the economics of capitated health care.

Because compensation affects behavior, it is critical that everyone who influences the delivery and cost of care understand the economics of capitated health care. Old measures of success under fee-for-service models will need to be discarded as new measures of success are implemented. For example, under fee-for-service reimbursement, hospital managers focused on achieving high occupancy rates. In a capitated environment, health care managers should strive to provide "the right care, the right procedure, in the right setting, in the right amount," which should produce lower hospital occupancy rates.[1] Success under capitation will be characterized by:

- Fewer hospitalizations
- Shortened hospital stays with improved efficiency of inpatient care
- Accelerated discharges from the hospital to other levels of care or the home through aggressive discharge planning and a truly coordinated continuum of care

Assessing Structural Readiness

Figure 1. Economics of Fee-for-Service Health Care

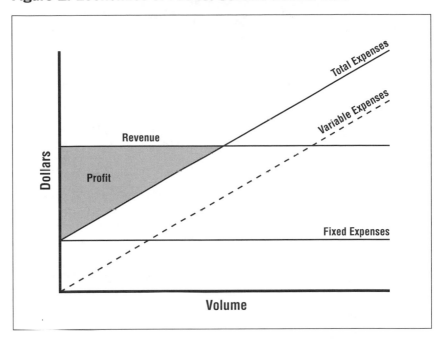

In addition to its effect on health care delivery, capitation has major implications for capital allocations. Board members need to understand capitation so that they can make prudent and appropriate capital allocation plans. Instead of continuing to invest in inpatient services, hospitals and boards should begin to develop a continuum of care and the infrastructure to support it. For example, major capital investments may be required to develop ambulatory or home care services to reduce length of stay.

On the other hand, an organization's most acute capital challenge may be the need to invest in information systems. Excellent information systems lessen the risk and uncertainty of capitated reimbursement. Information systems that feature cost accounting, track episodes of care, facilitate population-based analysis, and provide data to measure quality and outcomes will be especially helpful. It is important to remember, however, that board members will need to be prepared for the "sticker shock" associated with information systems designed for managing under capitation.

Board members, physicians, and staff also need to understand the positive features of capitation. Capitation changes the focus of health care from treating illness to promoting wellness and prevention. In addition, capitation aligns physicians' and hospitals' economic interests and thus allows the two providers to work as a team in developing ways to enhance quality of care and reduce costs of care. Capitation also provides a predictable revenue stream, based on enrollment.

Last, but not least, accepting capitation offers a health care organization

Figure 2. Economics of ~~Capitated~~ *FFS* Health Care

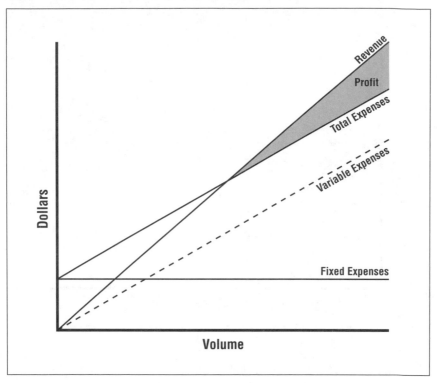

the opportunity to benefit financially from cost and care management. With risk can come reward!

What Is Needed to Answer Yes?

To answer yes, all providers of care must (1) acknowledge that capitation will be the predominant payment structure in the future and (2) be prepared to change their behavior accordingly. A basic understanding of capitation is evidenced by a provider's willingness to enter into a capitated contract or by a provider taking steps necessary to position an organization to enter into capitated contracts. An understanding of capitation is demonstrated by a proactive, not a reactive, attitude. Top-level management should ensure that all constituencies who influence the cost of care truly understand how capitation will change the way health care is delivered. For example, educational activities should be offered. In addition, "veterans" of capitation can be invited to share war stories with medical staff and board members.

Management should be prepared to offer several educational sessions and/or approaches to ensure that department directors, physicians, and board members truly understand capitation and recognize the behavioral changes needed for success. Providers must not only understand the reimbursement structure that exists under a capitated system, they must also understand how capitation will affect health care delivery. Only those organizations whose medical staff members, senior managers, department directors, and board members have a basic understanding of capitation should receive credit for this criterion.

What about Partial Credit?

Partial credit is not an option for this criterion. Without a basic understanding of capitation, providers of health care will be unwilling and unable to change the way they deliver health care to reflect the economic realities of capitation and succeed in a capitated environment.

Where Are Most Organizations Today?

Although many organizations have sponsored educational sessions and many individuals have been exposed to the principles of capitation, few organizations have truly adapted to the economics of capitation. The ultimate test of organizational adaptation is capital allocation, that is, putting the organization's money where its vision is. Most hospitals and systems sponsored by hospitals continue to invest the preponderance of their capital in hospital-based activities, including inpatient services.

Criterion 2

Structural Readiness	No	In Progress/ Needs Improvement	Yes
2. Top management emphasizes and rewards innovation and prudent risk taking.	0	0	1

Why Is the Rewarding of Innovation and Prudent Risk Taking Important?

Hospital managers (with the exception perhaps of some managers in proprietary organizations) historically have been risk averse. Most hospital managers have rewarded planning efforts based on extrapolation of historical trends, successful efforts at other facilities, and/or projections of financial payoffs in the early years of investment. However, historical experience is no longer a good predictor of success.

In 1993, the national average number of inpatient days for a population of 1,000 was 702.[2] For an HMO-enrolled population of 1,000, the average number of inpatient days was 465, and in selected California integrated systems the number was 238.[3,4] Once the transition to capitation occurs, the hospital that projects its need for beds based on historical use rate trends will have excess inpatient capacity and inadequate outpatient capabilities for health care delivery in a capitated environment. In addition, such organizations may expend all their capital resources on the development of inpatient capabilities and lack the capital required to restructure for success under capitation.

When a provider enters into a fee-for-service contract to provide health care, the provider assumes little or no financial risk. However, as payers move from a traditional contractual payment structure to a capitated structure, the amount of risk assumed by the provider increases. To succeed under capitation, organizations will have to accept prudent risk.

Prudent risk taking can be defined as understanding the implications of the risks an organization is assuming, distinguishing between risk and uncertainty, and being capable of managing the risk assumed. *Risk* implies that the probability of a loss or gain can be quantified or measured. For example, loss under a capitated contract may occur when an enrolled population consumes more health care resources than a provider estimated when developing its bid for the capitated contract. The risk of overutilization can be assessed through the use of actuarial data for similar populations.

Uncertainty results when management lacks complete knowledge of an issue, does not understand the "rules of the game," or fails to analyze a situation appropriately. For example, uncertainty occurs when management decides to bid on a contract just because a competitor is doing so, without knowing the risks and/or potential financial implications of the proposed contract.

Prudent risk taking has occurred when management has:

1. Identified the risks it will be assuming
2. Evaluated the potential financial implications of risk assumption
3. Developed systems and assigned responsibilities to manage risk
4. Taken appropriate actions to mitigate risks
5. Monitored the results of the contract/project
6. Taken appropriate actions to resolve differences between actual and anticipated results
7. Discontinued (if necessary) the contract/project after it has been determined that the risks assumed have resulted in greater-than-acceptable losses and after it has been decided that there is no remedy for the situation

What Is Needed to Answer Yes?

The structural readiness criterion specifies that management emphasizes and rewards innovation and prudent risk taking. Although it may be easy for management to espouse this concept, it must also be ready to act on it. Management that effectively emphasizes and rewards innovation and prudent risk taking must:

- Communicate the value of prudent risk taking and the financial rewards that will be realized by those who take risks
- Develop a compensation structure that rewards successful and prudent risk taking
- Allow people to make mistakes
- Support individuals who took prudent risks and whose projects were later discontinued

This philosophy is illustrated by one hospital administrator's statement: "Risk taking is part of taking the lead. Mistakes are going to happen in the first few years—they happened here, when we were new to capitation. Just go out there and get those contracts and make them work; you'll learn by doing, not by waiting."[5] Similarly, according to a California medical group administrator, "Every time we've had a tough time here [at the medical group], we've learned all kinds of new things. It's that old Nietzschean philosophy: 'What doesn't kill you makes you stronger.' "[6]

What about Partial Credit?

Partial credit is inappropriate for this criterion. Mixed messages cannot motivate people to behave in the desired manner. If innovation and prudent risk taking are valued by an organization, such initiatives cannot merely be allowed to occur; they must be acknowledged, promoted, and rewarded.

Criterion 3

Structural Readiness	No	In Progress/ Needs Improvement	Yes
3. Hospital/system has ownership of or tight contractual relationships with facilities and services to provide a full continuum of care (accounts for at least 90 percent of the nonprofessional costs of health care).	0	1	3

To succeed under capitation, a hospital or health care system must be able to deliver the most appropriate care in the most cost-effective setting. Meeting this challenge requires that the organization is prepared to provide a full continuum of care. A *full continuum of care* includes *health* services focused on health promotion and illness/injury prevention as well as *health care* services focused on the diagnosis and treatment of illnesses. Typically, a full continuum of care encompasses three different settings: ambulatory, inpatient, and home. Figure 3 provides a schematic representation of the continuum of care.

Why Is the Continuum of Care Essential under Capitation?

Capitated reimbursement takes the form of integrated payment. A provider system or network that accepts a global capitated payment is at financial risk for all services (except a few that may be "carved out" of the capitated payment) used by the enrolled population. A global capitated payment essentially is a budget maximum; regardless of overall utilization patterns and levels, the network receives no more than the capitated payment to cover its total costs.

Cost control is the most critical success factor under capitation. Without a tightly linked continuum of care, adequate cost control is difficult, if not impossible. A full continuum of care provides two important cost-management opportunities. Costs can be controlled through:

1. Substitution of less-costly types of treatment for more-expensive methods (for example, psychiatric partial hospitalization offered in lieu of inpatient care)
2. Management of resource consumption at each level along the continuum (for example, services provided at the right times in the right amounts)

Assessing Structural Readiness

Figure 3. Continuum of Care

Ambulatory Care		Inpatient Care			Home Care	
Prevention	Primary Care	Specialty Care	Acute Care	Subacute Care	Nursing Home Care	High-Tech Care	High-Touch Care
• Public health education • Immunization • Research • "Wellness" programs • Advocacy • Industrial health	• Physician care (medicine, pediatrics, obstetrics/ gynecology) • Routine outpatient diagnostics • Patient education • Urgent care centers	• Physician care • Ambulatory surgery • Imaging centers • Sports medicine • Outpatient rehabilitation centers • Adult day care	• General acute • Specialty — Women's health — Rehabilitation (short term) — Psychiatry — Ear, nose, and throat medicine — Orthope- dics/sports medicine — Substance abuse	• Surgical recovery centers • Rehabilitation (long term) • Brain injury centers • Birthing centers • Inpatient hospice care	• Skilled care • Intermediate care • Personal care • Alzheimer's units	• Durable medical equipment • Infusion therapy • Parenteral therapy	• Home health care • Home aides • Outpatient hospice care

Do You Have a Full Continuum of Care?

To evaluate the adequacy of your continuum of care, estimate how the average health care dollar is spent in your system. Table 1 shows how health care services might be segmented for such an analysis. Our rule of thumb for determining an adequate continuum of care is that you should control, either directly or indirectly, the services that together account for at least 90 cents of every dollar spent on nonphysician health care services. Although the services that account for the remaining 10 percent also need to be provided, each service will represent so little of your capitated budget that it will not be necessary to offer them yourself or negotiate formal contracts for them.

Based on table 1, your system should have at least the following components in its continuum of care in order to serve both commercially insured and Medicare-insured populations:

- Inpatient medical/surgical, psychiatric, and maternity services
- Skilled nursing and extended care services

Table 1. Sample Distribution of Health Care Spending

Type of Service	Percentage of Commercial Population Monthly Claims Cost	Percentage of Medicare Population Monthly Claims Cost
Inpatient		
Medical/surgical	38.5	49.2
Psychiatric	4.0	0.3
Alcohol/drug abuse	1.5	0.1
Maternity	11.3	0.0
Skilled nursing/extended care	0.1	4.8
Subtotal	55.4	54.4
Outpatient Hospital		
Emergency	6.5	2.3
Surgery	18.6	11.4
Radiology	8.0	4.1
Pathology	2.8	2.5
Maternity	0.5	0.0
Other	3.6	3.5
Subtotal	40.0	23.8
Other		
Home health/private duty nursing	1.5	16.5
Ambulance	1.1	1.6
Durable medical equipment	1.6	2.4
Prosthetics	0.4	1.3
Subtotal	4.6	21.8
Total	100.0	100.0

Note: This distribution excludes physician services and prescription drugs.
Source: Adapted from Milliman & Robertson's Commercial and Medicare Actuarial Models for Aggressively Managed Systems, published in *Integrated Healthcare Report*, Dec. 1994.

Assessing Structural Readiness

- Outpatient hospital services including a broad range of emergency services, outpatient surgical services, and radiology and laboratory services
- Home health care services

Our survey tool indicates that ownership of the full continuum of care is not necessary; in fact, it may be undesirable. Your hospital/system can focus its scarce resources on what it does best by partnering with other providers to fill gaps in the continuum of care. These other providers can offer the services for which they hold the competitive advantage. Ensuring the durability of partnership arrangements with other providers is the key to a full continuum of care. The following conditions are required for lasting partnerships:

- The partners pursue managed care contracting jointly. Specifically, they create a joint venture contracting vehicle and invest it with a right of first negotiation both for new contracts and existing contracts as they come up for renewal.
- The partners share financial risk for utilization decisions/resource consumption.

What Is Needed to Answer Yes?

The challenges associated with the provision of a full continuum of care typically are threefold:

1. Ensuring that the right mix of services is offered
2. Ensuring that the services are "sized" adequately to meet population needs and to support one another
3. Ensuring that the continuum of services functions like a system

An organization should answer yes to the continuum of care question only when it has the right services in the right amounts *and* these services are working together well. *Having the right services* means that the 90 percent test described in the preceding section has been met. *Having the right amounts* means that services are available when they are needed (for example, skilled nursing beds are available without delay to facilitate early discharge of patients from the hospital). Finally, *services working together* means that:

- There is some evidence that consumers/users perceive the continuum of care as a system.
- Staff members view themselves as working in a system of care.
- Patients are transferred to different levels of care easily and on a timely basis.
- Treatment plans are coordinated across the continuum (that is, clinical protocols or pathways have been developed for treatment across multiple settings/levels of care).

Criterion 3   **19**

- Information is compatible and flows readily from one level of care to another.

What about Partial Credit?

Organizations that answer no to the continuum of care question usually have not yet invested in the development of the right mix and scope of services along the continuum of care. Those that rate their efforts as "in progress/needs improvement" typically have taken steps to fill gaps along the continuum but either have not addressed all needs adequately or have not yet achieved a coordinated system of care.

Where Are Most Organizations Today?

Most hospitals and health care systems have made some progress in building a continuum of care, but they still have substantial work ahead of them to make the continuum function in a coordinated and efficient manner. We have seen many health care organizations shift their priorities from development of hospital services to development of other services along the continuum of care. However, most organizations have focused on building subacute and home health care services—services in the middle and on the far right-hand side of the continuum of care. Services on the far left-hand side of the continuum—prevention and health promotion services—also must be a priority for providers under capitation. Today, few resources are invested in developing or offering prevention and health promotion services precisely because the predominant form of payment, fee for service, does not reward providers who offer such services. Under capitation, significant financial rewards are available to health systems that promote health, thereby reducing the overall costs of health care.

Criterion 4

Structural Readiness	No	In Progress/ Needs Improvement	Yes
4. Hospital/system has a strong, tightly aligned, and geographically dispersed primary care base.	0	1	2

The advent of the role of primary care physician as a "gatekeeper" has made virtually every hospital and health care system in the United States understand the need to strengthen and develop its primary care base. Primary care professionals—including both physicians and so-called mid-level providers such as nurse practitioners, physicians' assistants, and nurse midwives—serve as the primary channel of distribution for integrated delivery systems/networks.

What Is an Effective Primary Care Base?

A primary care base must demonstrate the following three characteristics to support a health system effectively:

1. Adequate strength
2. Appropriate alignment among the physicians and between the physicians and the hospital/health system
3. Accessibility to the population served

These characteristics are discussed in the following subsections.

Strength

The first characteristic of an effective primary care base, strength, encompasses several qualities. The first of these qualities is an *adequate number of primary care physicians.*

Primary care physicians include those trained in and practicing general internal medicine, family practice, or general pediatrics. (Obstetricians/gynecologists are excluded from the usual definition of primary care physicians.) A typical rule of thumb for determining an adequate number of primary care physicians calls for 1 primary care physician for every 2,000 enrollees or residents served. This ratio will vary according to the age and sex mix of the population you serve. You can estimate the number of primary care physicians needed to support your hospital or system by using your organization's market share as a "proxy" for the share of residents who rely on your organization for their care.

For example, if you are located in a three-hospital community with approximately 350,000 residents in its service area and your current market share is 40 percent, your organization would need 70 affiliated full-time equivalent (FTE) primary care physicians (350,000 population x 0.40 market share x [1.0 FTE primary care physician ÷ 2,000 residents] = 70.0 FTEs).

Another quick way to ascertain whether your organization has an adequate number of primary care physicians to meet the demands of a capitated system is to calculate the ratio of primary care physicians to total physicians on the organization's medical staff and then compare your result to the managed care target of 50 percent. If your organization's ratio is at least 45 percent primary care physicians, you probably have an adequate number of primary care providers on staff.

In addition, your primary care physicians all should be board certified. Exceptions should be granted only for those physicians (typically family practitioners) who completed their residency training prior to the establishment of a board certification process for their specialty. However, any physician who completed training after 1989 should be required to achieve and maintain board certification.

The second quality associated with a strong primary care base is a *commitment to managing care and serving as a gatekeeper*. The economics of capitation require providers to change how health care is delivered. The primary care physician is the key to medical management (and financial survival) under capitation. In essence, the primary care physician who serves as a gatekeeper becomes a substitute for the off-site "1-800-" medical management and utilization review mechanisms currently in place.

Although many primary care physicians support the underlying principles of managed care and enthusiastically embrace their new role as gatekeeper, other primary care physicians resent capitation because it alters their relationships with specialist colleagues and/or because they believe their patients' interests will not be well served by the new system. A strong primary care base includes leaders who are committed to the gatekeeper role and willing to teach other physicians—both primary care physicians and specialists—how to implement an effective gatekeeper model.

A third quality associated with a strong primary care base is a *willingness to use mid-level practitioners* to expand the primary care base. There should be no reluctance to utilize a broader mix of professionals than physicians alone to provide primary care services. As mentioned earlier, these professionals can include nurse practitioners, physicians' assistants, and nurse midwives.

Alignment

Incentive systems that reward the delivery of high-quality, cost-effective care and that align incentives among primary care physicians *and* between the physicians and the hospital/health system are the second characteristic of an effective primary care base. Specifically, a tightly aligned primary care base should demonstrate the following features:

- *Primary care physicians share risk among themselves.* Primary care physicians should agree to share the economic risk associated with managing the care of a panel of enrollees, even if the physicians still practice independently. This risk-sharing approach increases the effectiveness of peer review because the performance of each physician can contribute to rewards for the whole.
- *At a minimum, primary care physicians contract jointly with the hospital.* It is desirable and perhaps essential for the hospital to establish a vehicle by which primary care physicians and the hospital jointly can negotiate contracts with insurers. One such vehicle is the physician–hospital organization (PHO), which typically includes specialists as well as primary care physicians. (Physician–hospital organizations are described under structural readiness criterion 10.)
- *Over time, primary care practices are integrated into the local health system.* Primary care physicians are opting out of private practice in many mature managed care markets across the United States. Young primary care physicians often look for "salaried" positions. Established physicians often are willing, if not eager, to sell their practices, and in some cases they are selling their practices to new "group practices" structured within their local health care system. There are numerous models for integrating primary care practices into the local health care system, including:
  - The *management services organization (MSO)* model, which typically provides all administrative services for the physicians and contracts on behalf of the physicians. In this model, the physician may maintain a separate professional corporation for himself or herself.
  - The *affiliated group practice* model, which typically is established as a professional corporation controlled through its sole corporate member (a physician who holds a position such as vice-president of medical affairs at the health system).
  - *Direct employment* of the physician, often in a "physician division" of the health care system.

Accessibility

The final characteristic of an effective primary care base is geographic accessibility to the population served. Referrals to specialists on a hospital's staff often originate from primary care physicians unknown to the hospital (that is, not on the medical staff). Yet these referrals may be essential to maintaining the critical mass of patients required for the delivery of high-quality and cost-effective care.

You can determine "where" primary care physicians are needed to support your overall health care system by using the physician-to-population ratio described earlier. Some of the physicians identified on the basis of geographic accessibility may be "new" to your system (for example, they may have a historical referral relationship with your specialists but hold admitting privileges elsewhere). If this is the case, it is essential that these physicians meet preestablished quality standards, as well as demonstrate commitment to and effectiveness in managing care.

What Is Needed to Answer Yes?

You should answer yes and score two points for this criterion if your hospital or system has met *at least* the following requirements:

- There is an adequate number of board-certified primary care physicians (as determined by the ratios described earlier), and they are appropriately distributed geographically.
- The primary care physicians have agreed to share risk among themselves.
- At a minimum, a joint contracting vehicle such as a PHO is in place in which all the primary care physicians participate, *or* the physicians are part of a hospital-sponsored MSO or group practice.
- The primary care physicians are committed to and have demonstrated their competence in performing the gatekeeper role.

What about Partial Credit?

If you currently are working on all four of the preceding requirements and expect these features to be in place within 18 months, you qualify for the "in progress/needs improvement" score of one point. Otherwise, no points can be awarded under this criterion.

This one criterion of the organizational readiness self-assessment tool is critical to the success of local health care systems in a capitated environment. Today there is tremendous competition for the loyalty of qualified primary care physicians who are willing and able to play the essential gatekeeper role. This competition not only comes from historical competitors such as other hospitals or hospital networks, but also finds its source in fiercely independent physician groups (often backed with venture capital), national physician management companies, and insurers. In order to win this competition for gatekeepers, hospital and health care system executives must:

- Overcome physician distrust of large organizations, especially specialist-dominated hospitals. Primary care physicians are inundated with information that supports their hesitation to integrate with a "bureaucracy" such as a hospital. In addition, many primary care physicians believe that historically hospital management has "preferred" specialists, and primary care physicians continue to be skeptical about how real and long-lasting the current shift in emphasis toward primary care will be. These physicians will expect and require continued, visible support from management in the upcoming political struggles with specialists over economics.

- Offer an innovative practice model designed to meet the needs of the physicians, *not* the needs of the system.
- Import practice management expertise. Hospitals generally have little experience managing physician practices efficiently. It is wise to acquire practice management support from outside sources because developing such expertise internally takes too much time.

Criterion 5

Structural Readiness	No	In Progress/ Needs Improvement	Yes
5. Physicians are actively involved in using case mix, cost, and quality information to improve hospital service delivery.	0	1	2

This criterion is multidimensional and differentiated from information readiness criteria 3, 7, 8, and 9 (which also address case mix, cost, and quality) by the key words *physicians are actively involved in using.* Physician involvement in using case mix, cost, and quality information can be viewed along a continuum, as shown in figure 4. Ideally, the hospital maintains the underlying information, and physicians are encouraged to ask questions about hospital performance and are given timely, open access to hospital data.

Why Is Physician Involvement Important under Capitation?

Although it is important to have effective information systems in place, such systems are worthwhile only when case mix, cost, and quality data are actively used. Hospital managers can analyze case mix, cost, and quality information to try to improve performance, but the largest performance improvements will occur when physicians contribute their insight and expertise to the analysis.

Figure 4. Continuum of Physician Involvement in Using Case Mix, Cost, and Quality Information

No Physician Activity		Limited Physician Activity		Extensive Physician Activity
a	b	c	d	e
Information is not available.	Hospital has some or all underlying information, but physicians do not see it.	Physicians receive periodic reports about themselves only.	Physicians participate on hospital-defined teams that focus on specific cases, and information is provided about those case types.	Physicians identify and follow through on opportunities to enhance hospital service delivery. Information is provided as requested by physicians.

What Is Needed to Answer Yes?

To score this criterion, first evaluate information readiness criteria 3, 7, 8, and 9. You must be able to respond yes to each of these information criteria in order to answer structural readiness criterion 5 with a yes. However, a yes response to the four underlying information criteria is not enough; case mix, cost, and quality data need to be linked to each other so that the effects of changes in one area (for example, cost) can be evaluated, measured, and monitored in the other areas (for example, quality). Also critical is *how* case mix, cost, and quality information is shared and used. Physician involvement in using this information to improve service delivery requires that physicians have access to the output of case mix, cost, and quality systems. Physicians also should be encouraged to question and explore health care delivery processes. If your hospital can be viewed as occupying area d or e in figure 4, and if your hospital can meet the previously mentioned requirements, then you can answer yes and score two points for this criterion.

What about Partial Credit?

The "in progress/needs improvement" score can be achieved if some of the underlying information systems are being developed or enhanced or if physician involvement in using the information is sporadic or passive. To score partial credit, there must be at least a case mix system in place (see information readiness criterion 8), so that physicians can explore care delivery processes for different case types. Physician exposure to case mix, quality, and cost information is also required to score one point. At a minimum, physicians must receive reports of their activity, which would place a hospital in area c on the physician-involvement continuum. If physician activity information is maintained by your hospital but not shared with physicians, you must answer no to this criterion.

Where Are Most Organizations Today?

Most hospitals have some of the building blocks in place for this criterion and fall into the "in progress/needs improvement" category. However, hospitals generally fall short of achieving this criterion in its fullest sense. Although many hospitals have adequate inpatient case mix systems, most have inadequate cost accounting and quality/outcome measurement systems.

Even hospitals that have the basic underlying information systems generally fail in creating an approach that results in physicians using the information to enhance service delivery. In some cases, physicians do not use the information because they feel that such efforts will take up too much of their limited time or inappropriately question the way that they provide care. In other cases, however, the hospital hoards its information because it is "proprietary" or because the hospital does not want physicians to engage in discussions that may be critical of the hospital's performance in providing timely or efficient health care services.

Criterion 6

Structural Readiness	No	In Progress/ Needs Improvement	Yes
6. Physicians and management work well together, and trust levels are high.	0	0	1

Why Is Trust Important?

Webster's Ninth New Collegiate Dictionary defines *trust* as the "assured reliance on the character, ability, strength, or truth of someone or something." Trust allows people to communicate openly and effectively; lack of trust makes communication difficult, if not impossible. As discussed in other sections of this book, capitation requires that hospitals and physicians establish collaborative arrangements to manage the costs of delivering care effectively. Capitation requires teamwork, and teamwork requires trust.

The risk sharing that occurs when physicians and hospitals share a single capitated payment makes hospital profits dependent on how well physicians manage care. Although hospitals also depend on physicians to manage care effectively under today's DRG payment system, under capitation, for the first time, physicians' incomes may be dependent on hospitals' efficiency and management as well. This financial interdependence requires a new level of trust between hospitals and physicians—trust in the ability of hospitals and physicians to achieve clinical excellence and cost efficiency and to share the financial consequences of clinical and/or cost inefficiency. Thus, trust is the primary foundation for successful hospital–physician partnerships under capitation.

What Is Needed to Answer Yes?

The following "essentials for trust" were proposed by one of our hospital clients. The factors should be considered before scoring this criterion. (The hospital shared these essentials with its physician leaders in the development of a vertically integrated delivery model.) These essentials for trust can be grouped into two major categories—competency issues and integrity issues. Competency issues concern the ability to deliver on promises made, and integrity issues refer to commitment to a set of values or a code of ethics. Ask yourself the following questions to assess the level of trust between/among constituencies in your organization:

- *Competency Issues*
  — Do the various constituencies have the skills necessary to perform their jobs effectively (for example, to meet defined objectives)?

— Do they have the resources necessary to perform their jobs efficiently (for example, in a timely and cost-effective manner)?
— Do they understand what is expected of them and have the capability to accomplish these tasks?
— Do they have the ability to solve/resolve problems and implement workable solutions?
— Can they identify, comprehend, and articulate their own interests and objectives, as well as those of others?

- *Integrity Issues*
   — Do the various constituencies have a desire and commitment to enter into trust-based relationships with each other?
   — Do they have a history of open communication, honesty, and truthfulness?
   — Do they acknowledge and deal openly with problems?
   — Do they handle conflict fairly?
   — Are they willing to accept responsibility and accountability?

The same hospital also identified the following impediments to trust, which can be categorized as (1) impediments inherent in any physician–hospital relationship and (2) impediments related to the specific individuals or organization(s). Inherent impediments are a "natural" result of the professional differences between physicians and hospitals (and even among physicians); organization-specific impediments are specifically related to management team and physician leader personalities:

- *Inherent Impediments*
   — Different training and knowledge bases
   — Different professional interests and objectives
   — Competition (for leadership control, hospital resources, patients, and so forth)
   — Continual changes in the health care environment
- *Organization-Specific Impediments*
   — Negative past experiences
   — Greed or dominant self-interest
   — Desire/need to control
   — Insecurity/fear
   — Lack of confidence in and/or respect for others

Consider your own hospital–physician relationships in light of the preceding issues and impediments. Organizations whose leaders can truly answer yes to at least three of the five preceding competency issues and at least three of the five preceding integrity issues should receive one point for this structural readiness criterion. No points are awarded for "in progress/needs improvement" responses. An organization that does not possess the essentials for trust will be unable to make progress on the other dimensions of capitation readiness.

Where Are Most Organizations Today?

Building trust among administrators and physicians can be particularly difficult given the cultural differences between the two groups. Physicians have been trained to work independently in an action-oriented manner, whereas hospital administrators generally have been trained to work in a more collaborative and deliberative manner. Moreover, hospital administrators and physicians have different organizational, political, and legal structures; different incentive systems; and different time horizons.[7]

Cultural differences concerning trust were apparent when our firm participated in a project to develop an integrated delivery system for a large hospital and its affiliated physicians. In one of the project's working sessions, the physicians cited several examples of the hospital withholding its business plans from medical staff members. In response, the hospital's CEO explained that he was disinclined to share strategic information with physicians because he felt the physicians might not maintain its confidentiality. The CEO's reluctance was based on his belief that hospital management has a fiduciary responsibility to protect the business interests of the hospital, whereas affiliated physicians have little to no such incentive. During these same working sessions, the physicians reluctantly revealed that they were in the process of establishing an independent practice association that could conceivably compete with the delivery system the hospital was working to form with these same physicians.

Although hospital administrators and physicians are likely to encounter many such obstacles in the trust-building process, trust-building efforts can create great rewards. Stephen Covey offers the following wisdom regarding trust: "Trust is the highest form of human motivation. It brings out the very best in people. But it takes time and patience, and it doesn't preclude the necessity to train and develop people so that their competency can rise to the level of that trust."[8]

In many cases, trust can be created by simply opening lines of communication. For example, physicians are empirically trained and typically respond well to quantitative data. The sharing of data between administrators and physicians can provide a base upon which trust may be built. Moreover, the mere act of sharing information (much of which may have been withheld in the past) demonstrates a commitment to building a long-lasting, mutually beneficial relationship.

As hospitals and physicians enter into capitated contracts and begin to share financial risks and rewards, the relationships between these two constituencies will be put to the test. Those partnerships built on a solid foundation of trust and mutual self-interest are most likely to succeed in the new managed care environment.

Criterion 7

Structural Readiness	No	In Progress/ Needs Improvement	Yes
7. Excellent concurrent review and utilization review functions are in place.	0	1	2

Why Are Review Functions Important?

Because the key to financial success under capitation is cost control and because the key to cost control is the effective management of health care services, review functions that monitor treatment patterns are critical. Numerous studies and headlines have reported on the amount of "unnecessary care" delivered in the United States and on differences in utilization among various geographic regions. For example:

- Milliman & Robertson, Inc., an actuarial and consulting firm, reported in 1994 that up to 59 percent of all patient days (days during which a patient was hospitalized) experienced by commercially insured people under age 65 may be unnecessary.[9]
- The Public Citizen Health Research Group reported that almost half of the 966,000 cesarean-sections performed in the United States in 1992 were unnecessary and added an extra $1.3 billion to national health care expenditures.[10]
- In 1986, the *Wall Street Journal* cited studies published in the *New England Journal of Medicine* and the *Journal of the American Medical Association* showing that:
  — In one part of Maine, 20 percent of women over age 74 had had a hysterectomy; in another part of the state, that figure soared to 70 percent.
  — Boston residents were half as likely to have had their tonsils removed as people in Springfield, Massachusetts, just 95 miles away.
  The *Wall Street Journal* article concluded that "how a given American is treated for a given ailment may depend on where he or she lives."[11]

Lack of standardization in health care delivery is one of the primary factors contributing to the high cost of services. It is also one of the factors that can be addressed in preparing for the cost-control initiatives necessary under capitation, which include the development of, and the monitoring of compliance with, clinical norms or standards of care. (See information readiness criterion 4.) Compliance with clinical norms or standards of care can be monitored through concurrent review and utilization review.

Concurrent review occurs while a patient is being actively treated (that is, the enrollee has become a patient and is receiving treatment at some point along the continuum of care within the integrated delivery system). Concurrent review can assess whether a patient is:

- Receiving care that is in compliance with clinical norms, standards, or protocols
- Receiving care at the appropriate point along the continuum (for example, whether the patient should be receiving care in an acute care setting or a rehabilitation setting)

Utilization review is an after-the-fact analysis of what happened to a patient. The goal of utilization review is to identify ways to improve treatment outcomes and efficiency.

What Is Needed to Answer Yes?

Effective concurrent review systems and utilization review systems reduce costs of care and demonstrate several key characteristics, including the following:

- All cases are reviewed within 24 hours of admission to determine the appropriateness of treatment in the inpatient setting. Preadmission certification occurs for all scheduled, elective admissions.
- Reviewers actively participate on the caregiving team by monitoring compliance with clinical pathways and identifying opportunities for improving quality and reducing cost.
- Review extends beyond the narrow focus of compliance with length-of-stay standards and examines resource consumption and management.
- Discharge planning/social work functions are integrated with concurrent review to identify and resolve any problems that may result in a longer hospital length of stay than is clinically appropriate. Barriers to discharging the patient to home or other settings are identified and addressed as necessary.
- The review process evaluates the cost-effectiveness of total patient care across the continuum of services, not just in the inpatient acute care setting.
- Problems or issues identified during the postdischarge utilization review process are discussed with the physician(s) involved, and preferred alternatives are identified.

Organizations whose concurrent review and utilization review functions exhibit all of the preceding features should answer yes and score two points for this criterion.

What about Partial Credit?

All hospitals have at least some precertification (concurrent review) and utilization review functions in place. If these functions are used only to ensure that third-party payers will compensate the hospital for its services or to determine the causes of negative patient outcomes, hospitals can score one point for this criterion. Organizations that lack any form of concurrent review and/or use retrospective review only sporadically should score a zero for this criterion.

Related Issues

Concurrent review functions and utilization review functions in capitated systems are designed to measure compliance with standards of care that have been shown to ensure high-quality outcomes while utilizing resources in an efficient manner. Effective review functions depend on the availability of clinical norms and the acceptance of those norms by the physicians and caregivers who are responsible for following them. Review functions are only one part of a broad clinical resource management system, the components of which include the information readiness criteria of this self-assessment tool. In addition, a comprehensive clinical resource management system should include the following:

- A medical director who is responsible for coordinating the development and adoption of clinical protocols and who works closely with or has responsibility for the utilization review function
- An admitting office staff that is knowledgeable about precertification standards and inpatient admission guidelines and is encouraged to question referrals that fall outside those guidelines
- A discharge planning team that at the time of admission works to identify where a patient is likely to go after an inpatient hospital stay and works to identify and overcome barriers to discharge to a less intensive or more appropriate setting
- A quality review and management function that can document a hospital's ability to deliver high-quality care (that is, care characterized by clinical quality and patient satisfaction) as the hospital works to control costs under capitation

Criterion 8

Structural Readiness	No	In Progress/ Needs Improvement	Yes
8. Interdepartmental cooperation is very good. The hospital uses a "team" approach and has moved away from a traditional (hierarchical) organization.	0	1	2

Why Is Interdepartmental Cooperation Important?

Cost control, the number one success factor under capitation, requires a team approach because no one individual or department controls the total cost of care delivery. The importance of a team approach is shown in table 2, which displays the results of an exercise in which management team members were asked to assess which of their organization's departments had the most influence over cost.

As demonstrated in table 2, average length of stay, which has a huge impact on health care delivery costs, may be affected by ancillary departments, operating room personnel, discharge planning, and admitting departments. The total average length of stay can be minimized by involving each of these departments in the delivery of care.

Table 2. Departments That Exercise the Greatest Influence on Hospital Costs

	Nursing Services	Ancillary Services	Operating Room	Discharge Planning/ Social Services	Central Services	Admitting	House-keeping
Length of Stay		X	X	X		X	
Room Costs	X						
Unit Cost of Ancillary Services		X			X		
Hospital-Acquired Infections	X	X	X		X		X
Cost of Non-chargeable Supplies	X				X		
Staffing Costs	X	X	X				

For example, controlling length of stay for an elective surgery begins with admitting and operating room scheduling. If there is a capacity problem in either the operating room or with postsurgical intensive care beds, elective admissions should be postponed. Elective patients should not be admitted to a hospital only to have their surgery delayed due to operating or postsurgical recovery capacity constraints. Likewise, all ancillary departments need to work together to streamline pre- and postoperative testing so that hospital stay is not lengthened by delays related to testing or required therapies. Finally, discharge planning should be involved from the time of admission to ensure hospital discharge is not delayed due to the unavailability of a nursing home bed or the failure to schedule required home health care services. Only when all departments work as a team can total length of hospital stay be reduced.

What Is Needed to Answer Yes?

For an organization to answer yes to this criterion, all of its members must work as a team and demonstrate a commitment to truly managing care. Hospitals that answer yes should no longer budget or evaluate departments as "profit centers." Team members must view themselves as cost centers and strive to reduce the cost of providing each episode of health care. The organization must routinely use multidepartmental teams to:

- Investigate ways to reduce staffing costs by:
  — Sharing and/or cross training staff as appropriate
  — Scheduling staff based on projected patient workloads
  — Using appropriate staff to perform required tasks (for example, using people other than registered nurses to perform basic care tasks)
- Improve communication and coordination among departments in order to eliminate:
  — Unnecessary delays in service delivery due to interdepartmental scheduling problems
  — Duplicated tests due to lost test results
  — Duplicated tests due to undocumented tests or test results
- Develop clinical pathways that ensure that care is provided:
  — In the right place (for example, providing outpatient and home health care instead of inpatient care)
  — In the right amount (for example, ensuring that tests and treatments are prescribed according to a patient's condition rather than according to outdated standing orders)

Successful teamwork can arise from individual initiative. For example:

1. A manager recognizes that his department's workload cannot justify the department's current staffing.
2. The manager identifies an opportunity for shared staffing with another department.

3. The manager contacts the department and negotiates resource sharing that results in a reduction of total staffing costs either for one department or for the two departments combined.

To promote true teamwork, management must develop congruent incentives among all constituencies that affect care decisions and cost of care. Management also must make a commitment to really managing care and modifying current patterns and/or methods of delivery. Traditional methods of care delivery are not necessarily appropriate in a capitated reimbursement setting. All care delivery should be reviewed, and ideas for improving the quality and efficiency of care should be explored.

What about Partial Credit?

Partial credit is appropriate for organizations that have begun to shift from a traditional (or hierarchical) philosophy to a team approach. This shift in organizational philosophy is evident when organizations no longer budget revenues at the departmental level. As long as an organization perceives its individual departments (laboratory or radiology, for example) to be profit centers, the organization does not warrant partial credit for this criterion.

Criterion 9

Structural Readiness	No	In Progress/ Needs Improvement	Yes
9. Hospital/system has the financial resources to absorb any start-up "losses" due to innovative contractual arrangements.	0	1	3

Why Are Financial Resources Important?

Under capitation, a contracting organization assumes financial risks from which its members were insulated in a fee-for-service environment. These risks include absorbing the potential adverse impact on costs of variations in frequency and intensity of services covered by the fixed rate negotiated for the contract.

Many changes are necessary for an organization to compete effectively under capitation. An organization must provide services across the full continuum of care (see structural readiness criterion 3) and across a broad geographic area (see structural readiness criterion 4). An organization also needs a contracting organization that is empowered to enter into risk contracts for all its members (see structural readiness criterion 10) in order to manage financial risks under capitation. In addition, an organization must be truly cost-effective in order to offer competitive prices while managing risks.

In parts of the country where capitation is prevalent, organizations are substituting less intensive services for more intensive services while still ensuring quality of care. For example, the number of patient days per 1,000 lives covered under a capitated contract is often less than one-third of rates for the population as a whole. Similarly, under capitation the use of ancillary services decreases, as do physician referrals. The use of subacute care, home health care, and/or outpatient rehabilitation services, however, often increases.

The organizational changes required for success under capitation cannot be accomplished instantaneously. For example:

- The creation of a geographically dispersed primary care network may require capital investment to develop sites and acquire physician practices.
- An organization can develop a full continuum of care by contracting/ aligning with other providers, but financing may be required to fill gaps in services.
- Information systems—the skeleton that supports the integrated organization—are enormously expensive to acquire/develop and implement.
- It takes time for newly integrated organizations to function effectively. New working relationships and power structures must be digested be-

fore significant cost savings are realized. An organization can iron out integration-related problems before pursuing capitation contracts, or it can buy into the market and then subsidize operations until efficiencies materialize. However, an organization that selects the former strategy risks being shut out of the market by the time the organization is ready to pursue contracts.

What Is Needed to Answer Yes?

If your contracting organization has free financial reserves (that is, monies not committed to other activities) to finance at least three and preferably five years of the types of transition activities previously cited, *and* the reserves are committed and truly available to your organization, you can answer yes and score three points for this criterion. The commitment and availability of financial reserves is a critical factor in scoring this criterion. Most contracting organizations are newly formed, and working relationships among partners are at an early stage of development. Consequently, most partners are very risk averse with respect to investing capital in assets and activities over which they have little control. The key question that must be answered is: "As an individual member of the contracting organization, am I willing to support an investment decision that could 'hurt' me but benefit the organization as a whole?" Unless the answer is an enthusiastic "Yes!" do not answer yes to this criterion.

What about Partial Credit?

If your contracting organization has one to three years of free reserves to finance transitional activities, *and* these resources are committed to the contracting organization, score one point under "in progress/needs improvement" for this criterion. Also, if your contracting organization has over three years of free financial reserves, but members of the organization have placed strong limitations on investing those monies (such as the contracting entity being able to invest a member organization's capital contribution only in activities under the direct control of that member organization), partial credit is warranted.

Unfortunately, most hospitals participating in contracting organizations are very parochial with regard to investing in activities that would make the contracting organization successful. As noted in the discussion of structural readiness criterion 2, hospital managers are generally risk averse and want reassurance that a venture has a high probability of success before investing hospital capital. However, in the current managed care environment, there is no such reassurance.

Assessing Structural Readiness

Criterion 10

Structural Readiness	No	In Progress/ Needs Improvement	Yes
10. The hospital and affiliated physicians have formed a contracting organization (for example, a PHO) that is legally and organizationally empowered to enter into risk contracts for all members.	0	1	3

Why Is a Joint Contracting Entity Important?

Managing under capitation requires teamwork between hospitals and physicians to control utilization and manage costs and care. A contracting organization such as a PHO can provide an effective structure for teamwork. Simply having a PHO in place is not sufficient, however. Using that PHO (or other joint contracting vehicle) to align the hospital's incentives and the physicians' incentives is imperative.

Having a contracting organization in place that can legally commit its members to risk contracts is critical in a rapidly evolving health care market. A PHO or similar vehicle empowered to contract on behalf of its members allows an organization to respond to the market quickly—or even to drive the market if members so desire.

What Is Needed to Answer Yes?

This structural readiness criterion specifies not only that a contracting organization must be in place, but also that the organization must be empowered to enter into risk contracts for its members. Although there is a legal rationale for wanting risk-sharing mechanisms in place, there are operational and structural reasons as well. Before an organization can share risk, it requires:

- Established membership criteria, which often incorporate economic credentialing principles based on efficiency of practice patterns in the hospital and, to the extent possible, in physicians' offices.
- Adopted performance targets or standards related to resource utilization, patient satisfaction, administrative compliance, and so forth.
- Agreement about rewards and penalties—most often financial—for compliance and noncompliance with adopted standards. That is, before sharing risk, an organization must agree to an incentive system that rewards desired behavior and "punishes," or at least does not reward, behaviors outside acceptable norms. The organization also must define those norms.

If all members of an organization have parallel incentives, and those incentives are congruent to the long-term viability of the organization, then the PHO should be successful in accepting and managing the risk associated with capitated contracts.

Organizations that have established a joint physician–hospital contracting vehicle with a predetermined set of rules for allocating capitated payments among its members, and with the ability to create and enforce parallel incentives and adherence to standards of care, should be credited with three points for this criterion. In addition, organizations that have established subpanels of physicians for risk contracting (even though not all PHO members are involved) may score three points for this criterion, as long as the previously listed factors are present.

What about Partial Credit?

Although many hospitals have formed, are forming, or are thinking about forming some sort of joint contracting entity with physicians, most of these entities are not ready to share risk. In many cases, hospitals and physicians approach the formation of joint contracting vehicles with a plan to move cautiously toward meaningful integration:

1. Establish an open PHO for which all physicians who meet some very basic licensure, practice, and geographic qualifications are eligible.
2. Agree on how to measure the value delivered by physicians.
3. Begin collecting the necessary data on member physicians' practices.
4. Set norms or standards.
5. Enforce the norms/standards, either by educating members whose practice patterns do not comply or by not renewing those physicians' PHO membership.
6. Determine the financial consequences for exceeding the norms/standards and for not meeting them.
7. Create an incentive system that will motivate everyone to strive to deliver *value*, that is, high quality at a cost the market will bear.

Although this process seems reasonable and logical in theory, political issues make it extremely difficult for an organization to narrow a panel that was created as "open."

You should score one point for this structural readiness criterion only if your organization has moved beyond the initial open membership stage and is beginning to measure performance and attempting to establish and enforce standards of care. For an organization to receive any score other than zero, its PHO must be able to commit members to contracts without having to ask each member whether he or she is willing to participate. If the PHO must still get the approval of individual physicians before committing them to a contract, give your organization a zero on this criterion.

Organizations that are still thinking about or even talking about the need for a joint physician–hospital contracting vehicle also should score no points. Intentions are good, but actions are needed to score points on this particular exam.

Where Are Most Organizations Today?

Many physicians and hospitals enter into discussions about PHO formation not to talk about sharing risk and capitation dollars but to create a defensive strategy and to answer the question, "How can we work together to slow the pace of change?" On the other hand, there are typically a few entrepreneurial physicians on any medical staff who see capitation as an opportunity to take control. Sometimes the physicians seek to set up their own networks (often focused on primary care), which may compete directly or indirectly with the contracting organization the hospital is trying to establish with its affiliated physicians. As risk sharing is not for everybody, so PHOs are not for everybody. Some of us put our money in certificates of deposit while others play the stock market.

Be sure to take time to educate your medical staff members about the managed care market, the rationale for forming a joint contracting vehicle, and the goals and objectives of the organization. In a recent study of PHO executives sponsored by Hamilton/KSA, *Hospitals & Health Networks*, and the American Association of Physician–Hospital Organizations, respondents identified "improving physicians' understanding of the health care market" as a main accomplishment of PHOs.[12]

Although risk sharing among physicians and between a hospital and select physicians is critical to success under capitation, the process required to reach a true state of risk sharing is time-consuming and perilous. Physician participation in the PHO development process is mandatory; shortcuts typically are unsuccessful. Finally, relationships between physicians and hospital managers need to be based on trust. Few people want to share financial risk with people they do not trust. As discussed under structural readiness criterion 6, lack of trust is a common stumbling block to successful partnerships.

Assessing Information Readiness

The following sections discuss the 10 information readiness criteria. Again, the importance of each criterion is explained, and then some or all of the following questions are answered for each:

- What is needed to answer yes?
- What about partial credit?
- Where are most organizations today?

Criterion 1

Information Readiness	No	In Progress/ Needs Improvement	Yes
1. Physicians can schedule patients and obtain results reporting directly via office computers.	0	1	2

Why Is Patient Scheduling and Results Reporting via Office Computer Important?

Because physicians directly or indirectly control the vast majority of health care costs, success under capitation depends on physician effectiveness and productivity. Furthermore, physician productivity and efficiency have a direct impact on hospital efficiency and patient satisfaction. Two aspects of health care service delivery especially affect physician effectiveness: scheduling patients and obtaining results.

Patient Scheduling

Treating patients on a timely basis when they require medical intervention achieves two major objectives. First, timely treatment elevates the health status of the covered population through the identification of medical problems at an early stage (and the possible prevention of problems altogether), which leads to lower health care costs that in turn can allow the physician and the contracting organization to be more competitive in pursuing capitated contracts. Second, timely treatment creates patient satisfaction, which is key to maintaining existing contracts and competing for new contracts. Dissatisfaction among a covered population can result in lost contracts, and lost contracts jeopardize the physician's individual practice and the viability of the contracting organization.

Physicians' use of computer scheduling can serve to increase hospital efficiency. For example, average staffing levels in ancillary departments can be decreased by using computers to better match staffing needs to departmental utilization and smooth the peaks and valleys of utilization. Furthermore, computerized scheduling allows for the simulation of patient admission flows to determine the most efficient scheduling of services (that is, a schedule that avoids bottlenecks and duplication of testing), which can result in shorter lengths of hospital stay.

In addition, an efficient scheduling system provides a number of benefits to patients. A frequent patient complaint is that the registration process is often confusing and difficult when various hospital services are being utilized (for example, a patient has to register as an outpatient after an inpatient stay). A well-designed scheduling system can avoid this aggravation and create high levels of patient satisfaction. Being able to communicate to a patient what to expect and when to expect it can reduce the trauma of a hospitalization or complex procedure and further enhance patient satisfaction.

Finally, an efficient, easy-to-use scheduling system is an attractive tool for physicians' office staff members. Also, staff members may demonstrate a preference for scheduling patients to receive services at a hospital that is linked by a computerized scheduling system. The bonding process facilitated by an effective scheduling system can help strengthen the relationship between physicians and the hospital.

Results Reporting

Cost-effectiveness is directly related to physician productivity. Innovations that help physicians treat patients more quickly while maintaining quality also allow physicians to see more patients. Such innovations, in effect, enhance throughput. Receiving results via computer reduces time loss associated with manual processing of medical records. In addition, a significant by-product of computerized results reporting is that data can be aggregated across physician practices and then used to develop profiles of best business practices.

Results reporting also can serve as the basis for productivity monitoring. For example, a results-reporting system could identify physicians who are ordering inappropriate or an excessive number of tests when compared to best-practice guidelines. Unnecessary duplication of tests can be avoided by sharing results (subject to patient confidentiality guidelines) throughout an integrated delivery system.

What Is Needed to Answer Yes?

If your contracting organization has a scheduling and reporting system in place that is used by at least 75 percent of the organization's active physician members, you can answer yes and score two points for this criterion. However, the system must be used actively, and physicians must be satisfied with the product and understand its use and potential.

What about Partial Credit?

If your contracting organization has a system in place that is used by 20 percent or more of active physician members, partial credit of one point should be scored for this criterion. However, partial credit should not be awarded if a system is in place but is used by fewer than 20 percent of active physicians.

Criterion 2

Information Readiness	No	In Progress/ Needs Improvement	Yes
2. Hospital/system is actively developing a database of current experience that links hospital, physician, and other affiliated providers' data to track services rendered to a patient throughout an "episode of care."	0	1	2

Why Is It Important to Track Services throughout an Episode of Care?

Structural readiness criterion 3 stressed the importance of offering a continuum of care. However, it was noted that it is not enough to have the pieces of a continuum in place; steps must be taken to ensure that the services are coordinated. A flexible and effective information system is an important tool for coordinating services along the continuum of care.

A hospital or health system that accepts a capitation payment must be able to track treatment throughout an entire episode of care to ensure high levels of quality and cost-effectiveness. An integrated database can contribute to such efforts by:

- Facilitating movement of patients within the continuum, thereby improving access to care
- Safeguarding against inappropriate care and unnecessary duplication of effort
- Generally improving communication among providers
- Providing practice pattern, cost, and outcome information

An integrated database can also improve operating efficiencies by reducing the paperwork burden for providers.

What Is an Episode of Care?

Webster's Ninth New Collegiate Dictionary defines *episode* as "an event that is distinctive and separate although part of a larger series." An episode of care typically is defined by a specific illness, injury, or course of treatment. An excellent example of an episode of care is care delivered to a pregnant woman. In this case, the episode of care generally begins with a positive pregnancy test and ends with a postpartum visit to the physician approximately six weeks after delivery. This episode encompasses care delivered in multiple settings by various providers, specifically:

- Regular prenatal exams provided in the physician's office
- Prenatal testing provided in either the physician's office or hospital outpatient departments
- Birth preparation/education classes provided in the hospital
- Inpatient care at the time of delivery
- Patient education on newborn care and breastfeeding provided in the hospital by nurses
- Home health care immediately following delivery
- Postpartum care provided in the physician's office

What Is Needed to Answer Yes?

According to Paul Henchey, director of business development for HBO & Company (a leading health care information systems company), all of the following requirements should be met for a hospital or system:

- Common identification numbers are used across the continuum for both patients and physicians.
- Standard data elements are collected across the continuum, including, at a minimum:
  — Name of primary care physician/gatekeeper
  — Name of ordering physician
  — Diagnosis codes (ICD-9-CM)
  — Procedure codes (CPT-4)
  — Charges
- The database is user-friendly; users across the system are comfortable using the database and feel that it "makes their lives easier."[13]

What about Partial Credit?

Partial credit is appropriate for hospitals/systems that have identified standard data elements and have begun collecting the necessary information at each site along the continuum even though their database may not yet be fully operational.

Where Are Most Organizations Today?

Today, most health care provider networks recognize the importance of tracking care across the continuum and have made some progress in doing so. The amount of progress made by these networks often depends on the following factors:
- How the network is structured (for example, as a loose alliance, a fully merged organization, or somewhere in-between)

- How long the network has been integrated
- How many sites/services the network is attempting to integrate[14]

Related Issues

One of the biggest challenges associated with tracking care across the continuum can be overcoming provider (particularly physician) resistance to sharing practice-related information.[15] Substantial time and effort may be needed to build the trust required to overcome this resistance. (See structural readiness criterion 6 for a discussion of building trust.)

In the future, an integrated continuum of care will be supported by much more sophisticated information systems than are available today. Such sophisticated systems will include electronic medical records and computerized clinical pathways, which are being developed in earnest. Current efforts to track treatment throughout episodes of care are a necessary first step in achieving the next generation of information systems to link the continuum of care.

Criterion 3

Information Readiness	No	In Progress/ Needs Improvement	Yes
3. A computerized quality/outcome measurement system is in place.	0	1	2

Today's computerized quality/outcome measurement systems fall into two broad categories: (1) severity adjustment systems that compare inpatient morbidity and mortality rates to those found in normative databases and (2) population-based systems that maintain a detailed profile of each enrollee. Such profiles report on enrollees' health status, prevention activities, medical record, and health encounter information.

Patient or enrollee satisfaction data, another important type of quality information, most often are gathered on an ad hoc basis and are not usually integrated into computerized systems. The National Committee for Quality Assurance (NCQA) is developing an annual member health care survey for managed care organizations, which is likely to create greater consistency in satisfaction measurement techniques and questions.

Hospitals typically have invested in severity adjustment systems, which can link with case mix and cost accounting systems to support clinical protocol development and assessment of the hospital's relative value (that is, quality of care and services versus cost). Managed care organizations and, increasingly, larger medical group practices have invested in population-based systems, which are becoming a necessary building block for managing capitated populations and generating information to comply with NCQA Standards of Accreditation for Managed Care Organizations.

Why Is Such a System Important under Capitation?

Under capitation, quality and outcome data are important for several reasons. First, as part of a hospital's internal capitation management efforts, these data can be linked with case mix and cost information to help ensure that acceptable patient outcomes are maintained while ways to decrease costs of care are explored. Quality and outcome data are also important components of quality assurance and physician credentialing efforts.

Furthermore, the development of quality/outcome measurement systems can enhance an organization's image and external marketing effectiveness. NCQA accreditation has become extremely important for managed care organizations. To the extent that a health care system's quality and outcomes data help a contracting managed care organization meet NCQA standards, the system's relationship with payers will improve. In addition, sophisticated payers are asking providers to supply such evidence of their quality and outcomes when negotiating contracts.

What is Needed to Answer Yes?

To answer yes and score two points for this criterion, a hospital must have a computerized severity adjustment system in place that has collected at least one year of historical data, as well as have a population-based system in place (although historical data may be minimal). The population-based system does not necessarily have to be maintained by the hospital; an affiliated entity such as a PHO may operate and maintain the system. In addition, to answer yes, the hospital and physicians must believe that the system's output is credible, and they must be willing to use the information in making decisions. Although computerized patient/enrollee satisfaction information is desirable, it is not required to answer yes.

What about Partial Credit?

To score one point under "in progress/needs improvement" for this criterion, a hospital must be in one of several possible stages of implementing a computerized quality/outcome measurement system. For example:

- A severity adjustment system is in place, but only limited historical data are available. A population-based system may or may not be in place.
- A population-based system is in place, but there is no severity adjustment system.
- A severity adjustment and/or population-based system is in place, but key constituents (for example, physicians) are not yet confident that the output is valid.
- A severity adjustment and/or population-based system is in place and has physician support, but the system is not computerized.

Where Are Most Organizations Today?

Some states have mandated the use of severity/outcome systems. However, acceptance and use of these systems vary considerably among hospitals. Some hospitals view the development of severity/outcome systems as merely a regulatory requirement and do not use output from the systems for any strategic purposes. Other hospitals tap into the information to examine clinical performance.

Outside of states that mandate severity/outcome systems, there is also significant variation among hospitals regarding investment in computerized quality/outcome systems. In many instances, a hospital's decision of whether and how to invest in this area is strongly influenced by a medical director or other medical leadership.

Related Issues

A hospital can view itself as a stand-alone facility or as a member of a system when deciding what kind of quality/outcome measurement system is most appropriate. For a hospital, a traditional inpatient-oriented severity/outcome system can support the management of risk under a hospital capitation or per-case payment. As a participant in an integrated delivery system, however, a hospital will need to invest (along with its partners) in a population-based system that not only measures the quality/outcome of a particular episode of care but also measures the health status of a capitated population. In addition, in the long term, development of a member-satisfaction measurement system will be critical to ongoing marketing and service improvement efforts.

Criterion 4

Information Readiness	No	In Progress/ Needs Improvement	Yes
4. Clinical protocols or norms are established and monitored for selected procedures/cases.	0	1	2

What Are Clinical Protocols?

Clinical protocols profile a course of treatment or the typical clinical path for a particular case type or certain types of diagnoses. Clinical protocols are also referred to frequently as *guidelines, care paths, pathways,* or *standards.* Hospitals, physicians, medical societies, managed care organizations, actuarial firms, and regulatory agencies are among the many groups that actively develop clinical protocols. The federal Agency for Health Care Policy and Research has published over 15 sets of guidelines since 1992. These guidelines cover a variety of conditions including unstable angina, acute lower-back problems, and otitis media. In addition, Milliman & Robertson (M&R), Inc., has developed the *M&R Healthcare Management Guidelines,* a collection of practice guidelines that have been adopted by many managed care organizations.

Many of these protocols or guidelines have been designed for very prevalent conditions (that is, conditions that have a high frequency of occurrence among a given population), which may or may not mean that the conditions require inpatient hospitalization. Hospitals often are most interested in protocols that focus extensively on clinical treatment during an inpatient stay. These inpatient protocols go beyond a simple expectation regarding length of stay. Inpatient case protocols should define expected treatment activities by day of stay. Figure 5 (pp. 52–53) shows a sample inpatient case protocol for DRG 107.

Upon establishment of a clinical protocol, performance compared to the protocol must be monitored, and reasons for variance from the protocol must be documented. Figure 6 (p. 54) shows an example of a monitoring report that summarizes the reasons for length-of-stay variances from protocols and lists the frequency of each reason.

Why Are Protocols Important under Capitation?

Clinical protocols are an extremely useful tool in managing costs of care while ensuring that appropriate treatment patterns are maintained. Such protocols are as useful under capitation as they are for case-based pricing systems (for example, DRG payments). Clinical protocols also can facilitate the utilization management process by providing a baseline against which to identify outlier patients who may require close case management and/or physicians whose prac-

Figure 5. Example of an Inpatient Case Protocol

Activity	Presurgery Visit	Day of Surgery	Day 1	Day 2	Day 3	Day 4
Visits	Surgeon Anesthesia Social services Physician's assistant Mended Hearts	Surgeon	Surgeon Physician's assistant	Surgeon Physician's assistant	Surgeon Physician's assistant	Surgeon Physician's assistant
Tests	Lab work X rays CXR-PA & LAT Chem 7, U/A EKG		EKG, CXR, Chem 7, CBC		CUC, Chem 7, CXR	
Activity	Out of bed ad lib	Pre-op bed rest Transported to OR Holding area on schedule ICU dangle ft. 4 hrs. post extub.	Dangle feet➝ to chair, 20 min. 2x/day Ambulate 50–100 ft.	Chair, 3x/day for 20 min. Ambulate 100–200 ft. a.m./p.m. Shower	Ambulate 100–200 ft. a.m./p.m. Stairs Evaluate outpatient rehab.	Patient discharged
Treatment/ care	Betadine shower	OR: prep. invasive lines ICU: Extubate/ maintain O_2	D/C Foley, Tri Lumen, CTs Telemetry Check incisions	Wean from oxygen Check incisions— clean and dry D/C pacing wires/Telemetry		

52   *Assessing Information Readiness*

Diet	NPO post MN except for specific needs	OR: NPO, I/O ICU: NPO until extubated, then ice chips	Liquids ➜ cardiac diet	Cardiac diet	Cardiac diet
Medications	D/C ASA, Coumadin, Incocin Routine meds per MD order	OR: Anesthesia ICU: If needed, inotropes, vasodilators, antiarrhythmiacs Anagesics	Aspirin Analgesics Adjust P/O meds	Pain meds Evaluate home meds regime	Review home meds on rounds Give pt. med list and prescriptions
Discharge planning	Discharge needs assessed Discharge planner/ social service involved with complex discharge		Transfer to cardiac telemetry unit Discharge planner & social service assess discharge needs	Discharge planner & social service & RN communicate D/C plan on rounds	Discharge plan complete
Teaching	Pre-op booklet given by RN PA reviews anatomy and surgical changes in anatomy	CVOR RN meets patient, explains process, provides support Post-op family teaching	Patient education checklist activated Begin patient teaching	RN confirms previous teaching	Attends discharge class RN reviews "survival skills," med card, follow-up appointments, and gives to family

Source: The Virginia Heart Center at Fairfax Hospital, Falls Church, VA.

Figure 6. Example of a Clinical Protocol Length-of-Stay Variance Report

Cause of Variance	Pre-op		Post-op	
	Reason	#	Reason	#
Patient condition	Work-up	1	Weakness	2
	Other	2	Other	4
			Observation	2
			Hypotension	2
			Arrhythmia	8
			A-Fib	5
			Infection	1
			Renal	3
			GI	1
			Cardiac	3
			Pulmonary	2
			Fever	1
Clinician	Transfers	8		
Hospital	OR	1		
Community				
	Total	12		34

Source: The Virginia Heart Center at Fairfax Hospital, Falls Church, VA.

tice patterns consistently differ from the protocols. In addition, the clinical protocol development process can enhance discussions of best demonstrated practice among physicians who treat patients with a given condition. Such discussions are particularly enhanced when protocols are developed from the ground up internally or when externally developed protocols have been used as a starting point and then modified internally by the organization.

What Is Needed to Answer Yes?

To respond yes to this criterion and score two points, your hospital should have protocols that are accepted and supported by physicians for at least 15 high-volume or high-cost case types. Patient medical records should incorporate the protocols, and exceptions to the protocols should be documented in the medical records. In addition, to answer yes, variance from protocols should be monitored, and attention should be paid to the number of patients falling outside of a protocol and the reasons why actual treatment did not follow a protocol.

What about Partial Credit?

A hospital must have at least five actively used protocols for high-volume or high-cost cases to score one point under "in progress/needs improvement."

Partial credit may be awarded if a hospital has more protocols but has not yet integrated the use of those protocols into the medical record or if a hospital has protocols but does not monitor and explore reasons for variance from protocols.

Where Are Most Organizations Today?

Many hospitals have some protocols or are beginning to adapt protocols from publicly available sources. Physician acceptance of protocols varies, ranging from enthusiastic endorsement to strong rejection.

Criterion 5

Information Readiness	No	In Progress/ Needs Improvement	Yes
5. Employer group and specific insurance plan are coded and accessible for all patients.	0	0	1

Why Is Payer and Employer Coding Important?

A contracting organization that is able to identify the payer and employer for each of its patients (or covered lives) can develop a comprehensive understanding of its relationship with its revenue sources, especially if the organization's information system has a good flexible report writer (see information readiness criterion 9). Specifically, payer data are important for the following reasons:

- Payer data reveal the extent of a contracting organization's dependency on individual payers, thus revealing how important a particular payer is to the organization's viability. Further, payer data can reveal whether a payer's covered lives are served by a concentration of a few providers within the contracting organization's membership or whether the covered lives are served by many providers throughout the organization. Such concrete information can help management focus marketing efforts on areas where the efforts can be expected to do the most good.
- Payer/employer identification data coupled with a product cost accounting system (see information readiness criterion 7) can reveal how profitable an organization's contracts are. This profitability information is critically important to contract renegotiation; an organization armed with hard data is more credible during renegotiation processes with payers or self-insured employers.
- Payer identification data coupled with a case mix system (see information readiness criterion 8) can reveal whether the resource consumption profile that served as the basis for the contractual agreement is still valid. A profile may become invalid for several reasons:
  - *Inappropriate internal controls:* For example, there is evidence of excessive or inappropriate referrals or consultations.
  - *Adverse selection:* The age/sex/demographics/health status of the covered population is different from that represented in contract negotiations.
  - *Structural "defects" in the contract:* Such defects can include first-dollar coverage, which encourages excessive demand for services by covered members, or incongruent referral incentives among

partners to the contract, which result in inappropriate utilization of physician services.

- Payer identification data coupled with physician-specific case mix/cost accounting data can reveal variations in profitability and resource consumption among physicians serving a particular contract. Such data can serve as the first step in diagnosing whether structural defects are present in a contract. (For example, an organization that provides primary care "profitably" and specialty care "unprofitably" within a particular contract should carefully investigate why such differences exist.)
- Employer identification data can reveal utilization trends and health care consumption patterns for specific employer groups. Such information can be used in discussions with self-insured employers (or their third-party administrators) to help the employers better understand and manage health care costs.

What Is Needed to Answer Yes?

If your contracting organization's information system database contains a payer field and an employer field for each patient (covered life) record *and* the information in each of the fields is accurate, answer yes and score one point for this criterion.

What about Partial Credit?

If your organization's information system database contains fields for payer and employer data, but payer and/or employer data are not recorded completely for each patient or the data's accuracy is questionable, you would fall into the "in progress/needs improvement" category. However, no points are awarded for partial credit under this criterion because of the importance of complete and accurate payer data.

Criterion 6

Information Readiness	No	In Progress/ Needs Improvement	Yes
6. Information system provides up-to-date tracking of which managed care plans physicians participate in.	0	1	2

Why Is Tracking Physician Participation in Managed Care Important?

Tracking physician participation in managed care allows hospitals to identify physicians who have successfully established strong managed care relationships in their practices. "Managed care–friendly" physicians are most likely to be approached for capitated contracts and are most capable of managing them. Furthermore, if a hospital's tracking system can identify payment methodology by physician (that is, fee schedule, capitation, and so forth), the hospital can identify physicians who already have capitation experience.

A tracking system also allows a hospital and its affiliated physicians to emphasize existing contracting relationships with managed care companies when contracts are being renegotiated. A managed care plan will favor capitation proposals from organizations that can show that a large number of their affiliated physicians have already contracted with the plan.

A third reason to track physician participation in managed care is to determine whether hospital-affiliated physicians provide adequate geographic and specialty coverage for each major area health plan. For example, tracking physician participation in managed care may help a hospital to recognize a shortage of contracted primary care physicians in a key geographic area. Finally, such a tracking system can be used to identify health plans with which a large number of physicians are contracted but the hospital is not.

What Is Needed to Answer Yes?

At a minimum, a managed care participation tracking system should include active physicians on the medical staff or in the PHO, but ideally an effective tracking system includes every medical staff physician. The primary information source for a tracking system database is managed care companies, not physician offices, because most physician offices are poor sources of up-to-date payer data and because it is easier to update data from 30 managed care companies than from 300 physicians' offices. In most hospitals, the department that maintains the tracking system will be the managed care department or the business office, not the medical staff department. Because managed care relationships change quickly, data must be updated at least quarterly. Finally, the tracking system should be tested for internal consistency with other organizational databases such as those found in the medical staff and financial departments.

To answer yes and score two points for this criterion, your tracking system database should meet the preceding requirements and contain the following data fields:

- Identification information for each physician:
  — Physician's name
  — License number (for common identification with managed care companies)
  — Medical staff number (for internal consistency with other hospital databases)
  — Specialty(ies)
  — Board certification status
  — Group affiliation
  — Office location(s)
  — Practice status (whether practice is open to new patients and whether restrictions exist)
- Managed care plan identification information for each area plan:
  — Plan name
     Plan type (HMO, PPO, POS, other)
  — Number of area covered lives
  — Hospital contract type (per diem, discount fee for service, capitation, none)
- Contract information for each physician, by plan:
  — Initial contract date
  — Contract expiration date
  — Payment type (discount from charges, fee schedule, capitation)

When basic physician and managed care plan data are combined in one database, standard reports that provide an overview of contract-related information by plan or by physician can be created. (Examples of standard reports are shown in figures 7 and 8, pp. 60 and 61.) In addition to standard reports, a tracking system should be able to produce ad hoc reports sorted by any of the fields in the preceding list.

What about Partial Credit?

Most hospitals do not have systems that track physician participation in managed care. Hospitals that have begun to track managed care participation on a limited basis should score one point for this information readiness criterion. Examples of tracking systems that warrant partial credit as in progress but need improvement include the following:
- Databases that contain fewer than 8 of the 15 previously listed data fields

- Databases that are updated annually or semiannually
- Databases that track "key" physicians only
- Databases that contain managed care plan data for hospital-contracted plans only
- Databases that are made up of incomplete data collected through physician offices and/or hospital records

Figure 7. Sample Managed Care Plan Report

Managed Care Plan Report

Plan Name: _____

Plan Type (HMO, PPO, POS, etc.): _____

Area Covered Lives: _____

Hospital Contract Type (Per Diem, Discount FFS, Capitation, None): _____

_____

Participating Physicians

Physician Name	License Number	Specialty	Date Contracted	Contract Expiration Date	Payment Type	Office Location(s)
1						
2						
3						
4						

Assessing Information Readiness

Figure 8. Sample Physician Managed Care Report

Physician Managed Care Report

Physician Name: _____

License Number: _____

Medical Staff Number: _____

Board Certification Status: _____

Specialty(ies): _____

Group Affiliation: _____

Office Location(s): _____

Practice Open/Closed/Restrictions: _____

_____

Contracted Managed Care Plans

Plan Name	Plan Type	Covered Lives	Date Contracted	Contract Expiration Date	Payment Type
1					
2					
3					
4					

Criterion 7

Information Readiness	No	In Progress/ Needs Improvement	Yes
7. A cost accounting system provides accurate fixed, variable, and total costs at a procedure level, which then can be aggregated to a patient case.	0	1	3

Why Is a Cost Accounting System Important?

Under a capitated contract, a health care organization's revenue depends solely on the number of covered lives, not on the actual frequency or amount of service rendered. Therefore, as is stressed throughout this self-assessment, to succeed under capitation, an organization must manage its costs effectively. An organization's ability to manage costs effectively can be enhanced greatly by a cost accounting system that calculates the fixed and variable costs of providing care to covered lives and that, through case mix analysis, decomposes any variance from expected cost into specific causes.

Information readiness criterion 7 focuses on an organization's ability to develop the building blocks for accurate cost information. In a hospital, total costs equal procedure-level costs (which are often determined by hospital management) times the number of procedures undertaken or produced (which is influenced to a great extent by physicians). Therefore, hospital management and physicians affect the total cost of providing care in a hospital. Hospital management is primarily responsible for *unit costs,* that is, the cost to perform a laboratory test or a specific procedure. Physicians have the greatest influence over the volume of procedures performed. Cost accounting systems, especially those linked with case mix systems, can analyze effectively the physician- and management-related costs of providing patient care.

What Is a Cost Accounting System?

A cost accounting system enables an organization to estimate the cost of a particular product by determining and aggregating the costs of the various input factors required to produce that product. In health care, the product in question is typically an inpatient or outpatient case. To estimate the cost of a patient case, the costs of the most basic units of service, for example, departmental procedures, tests, and exams, must be determined. These procedure-level costs then can be aggregated on the basis of the number and mix of procedures associated with a patient case.

Most hospital cost accounting systems also can perform case mix analyses that examine costs associated with specific groupings of cases. (Case mix systems and analyses are discussed under the next criterion.)

Cost accounting regularly occurs within each hospital department or cost center at an expense line-item level (for example, supply costs in the radiology department). A cost accounting system is required to determine costs at a procedural level within a department (for example, total salary costs associated with a three-view ankle X ray). The cost accounting process is made up of three major steps:

1. *Identify the cost categories to be maintained.* At a minimum, costs should be divided into salary, nonsalary, and capital-related costs. Although costs can be defined at a greater level of detail (for example, salaries by staff position), the incremental improvement in accuracy of the cost estimate of the end product usually is not significant enough to warrant this additional detail. In addition, line-item costs within each department should be categorized as fixed, variable, or a combination of fixed and variable. Cost accounting systems should be able to identify and maintain all categories of costs at a procedural, departmental, and patient-case level.

2. *Allocate costs in non–patient care departments to patient care departments.* For example, determine how accounting, admitting, and housekeeping costs should be allocated to nursing units and ancillary departments. This allocation process may be similar to the cost step-down procedure required to complete the Medicare cost report. However, the allocation bases may be different. For internal cost accounting, management should develop overhead allocation algorithms or methodologies that best reflect how costs accrue. Such algorithms may be significantly different from the Medicare allocation standards.

3. *Allocate department costs to individual procedures.* Relative value units (RVUs) that reflect the relative resource consumption of each procedure and that can be used as the basis for allocating department costs to individual procedures should be developed. A procedure-level RVU should be calculated for each cost category (that is, for salary, nonsalary, and capital-related costs).

Table 3 shows a cost accounting system report that lists the fixed and variable costs for a particular procedure (laboratory test ABC). Costs within the laboratory department and allocated costs from other departments are provided and categorized as salary, nonsalary, and capital-related costs.

Table 4 shows an example of an end product of a cost accounting system—a report of costs on a per case basis. In this report, fixed and variable costs are presented for DRG 162, Inguinal & Femoral Hernia. The cost accounting system determines the cost for this case type by summing the individual costs of all the procedures utilized in the patient cases within DRG 162. Reports listing costs and profitability by payer and case type are provided under the next criterion, which discusses case mix systems.

What Is Needed to Answer Yes?

Because cost accounting systems enable health care organizations to analyze alternative pricing strategies, clinical productivity initiatives, and the profitability of managed care plans in a capitated environment, cost accounting has become one of the most important tools available to health care management. The critical importance of a cost accounting system is reflected by the three points awarded for a positive response to this criterion.

To answer yes to information readiness criterion 7, an organization must have completed the three-step cost accounting process previously described and must be able to generate reports like those found in tables 3 and 4. In addition, all of the following conditions must exist:

- Physicians and department managers have been educated on cost accounting and have been involved actively in the development of underlying cost accounting data (for example, identification of fixed and variable costs and development of RVUs).
- Department managers receive and review department and procedure-level cost accounting reports on a regular basis.
- Cost accounting data are updated at least quarterly.
- The hospital uses a nurse acuity system to develop the RVUs for inpatient nursing care.
- Nursing unit and ancillary costs are captured by day of stay in recognition of the fact that utilization of services and therefore costs in the latter days of a patient's stay are usually less than those incurred during the first day or two.
- Hospital-specific RVUs have been developed, or industry standards (such as College of American Pathologists [CAP] units for laboratory

Table 3. Procedure-Level Cost Detail for Laboratory Test ABC

Cost Category	Laboratory Department Costs			Allocated Costs from Other Departments			Total Costs		
	Fixed	Variable	Total	Fixed	Variable	Total	Fixed	Variable	Total
Salary	$3.19	$0.00	$3.19	$0.67	$0.02	$0.69	$3.86	$0.02	$3.88
Nonsalary	0.70	0.91	1.61	3.55	0.07	3.62	4.26	0.98	5.24
Capital	0.00	0.00	0.00	0.36	0.00	0.36	0.36	0.00	0.36
Total test ABC	$3.89	$0.91	$4.80	$4.58	$0.09	$4.67	$8.48	$1.00	$9.48

Table 4. Cost Analysis of DRG 162 (Inguinal & Femoral Hernia)

	Fixed	Variable	Total
Cost for 55 cases	$75,292	$92,570	$167,862
Average cost per case	$ 1,369	$ 1,683	$ 3,052

costs) are used. (Using a departmental ratio-of-costs-to-charges process to allocate/determine costs does *not* satisfy this requirement.) In addition, separate RVUs are used for salary, nonsalary, and capital-related costs.

However, an expensive, time-consuming management engineering study does not have to be undertaken for each department in order to develop appropriate RVUs or to answer yes for this criterion. The 80–20 rule and work-sampling techniques can be used to develop RVUs for the procedures that represent the vast majority of a hospital's activities or costs.

- Outpatient cost accounting data are captured and used by the cost accounting system.
- The methodology for allocating fixed costs and non–patient care department costs to the procedure or case level is based on careful and ongoing study.

What about Partial Credit?

One point should be scored if an organization has completed the three-step cost accounting process previously described and is able to generate reports similar to those found in tables 3 and 4. In addition, at least four of the conditions in the preceding list must be true for the organization. Simply "having a system" is not sufficient to score partial credit.

Where Are Most Organizations Today?

A 1993 article identified four stages of cost accounting system sophistication and stated that many hospitals had not yet reached the first stage—the ability to determine the costs incurred by individual patients and patient groups, especially in outpatient service areas.[16] There seems to have been only minor improvement in this ability in recent years. In addition, those hospitals in which management indicates that a cost accounting system is in place usually have not met all of the previously identified conditions necessary to answer yes to this criterion. There are probably very few hospitals that deserve full credit.

Related Issues

There has been much debate regarding the need for and value of cost accounting systems ever since the first such systems were implemented in hospitals in the mid-1980s. Financial managers in hospitals that receive per-diem, per-case, or capitated payments have sometimes argued that procedure-level charges and costs are irrelevant. However, in general, costs must be identified at the procedure level in order to develop a "more useful" product-level cost (for example, cost per case or day). On the other hand, there are certain costs that are only relevant at a case level and do not need to be allocated to the procedure level (for example, admitting department costs).

Criterion 7   **65**

People who doubt the value of cost accounting systems have often argued that because a large portion of a hospital's costs are fixed, reducing total costs is the best way to achieve economic gains under capitation. Therefore, the critics maintain, the level of detail provided by a cost accounting system is unnecessary.

However, cost accounting systems can affect a hospital's economic gains in at least two ways under capitation:

1. Although hospitals must reduce the portion of their costs that is fixed, hospitals also should begin to manage their costs as if a greater portion of them were variable. Close cost management is critical under capitation because large portions of a hospital's business could disappear with the loss of a managed care contract.
2. One of the most important applications of a cost accounting and case mix system is analysis of where and why costs are different than expected/budgeted under a capitated contract.[17] The detail provided by a cost accounting system is necessary to analyze such variances.

Cost accounting systems will become more sophisticated as capitation contracts become more common and as more hospitals join integrated delivery systems. In the future, one of the most difficult challenges will be the development of cost accounting systems across multiple sites for the full continuum of services, including inpatient and outpatient services, home care, long-term care, physician office services, and other ambulatory care center services.

Criterion 8

Information Readiness	No	In Progress/ Needs Improvement	Yes
8. A case mix system provides volumes, payment amounts, and costs (if available) by procedure, DRG, physician, payer, day of stay, and so forth.	0	1	2

Why Are Case Mix Systems Important?

A case mix system enables a hospital to profile the types of patients treated and the services or resources actually used in treating those patients. In addition, a case mix system enables a hospital to determine whether the expected number of cases within a particular disease category actually occurred.

For example, Hospital XYZ has a capitated contract for 20,000 covered lives, and in an average population of 20,000 people, 80 inpatient diagnostic cardiac catheterizations are expected annually. A case mix system easily can determine the number of catheterizations performed on patients covered by Hospital XYZ's capitated contract and can provide supporting information to profile the patients and the primary care physicians and cardiologists involved in their care. However, a case mix system cannot provide management with reasons for any variance from an expected number of cases.

Physician-specific data are critical to hospitals as they manage their costs under capitation. Utilization and resource consumption by physician, as well as physicians' adherence to clinical guidelines, can be analyzed with a case mix system. Physician-level data also are essential as organizations such as PHOs implement economic credentialing or develop subpanels of physicians based on "performance." If a case mix system is linked to a clinical outcomes measurement system or patient satisfaction database, clinical outcome and patient satisfaction indicators also can be used to identify the "best" physicians.

What Is a Case Mix System?

A case mix system enables hospital management to examine utilization, payments, and costs (if a cost accounting system is in place) at the patient case level or any aggregation thereof. Patient cases typically are aggregated by diagnosis (for example, by DRG), by procedure, by ambulatory patient grouping, by payer, or by physician. Groupings of case types, however, can be based on any data element that is recorded as part of standard patient case information, including, for example:

- Patient age cohort
- Severity of illness within a particular diagnosis
- Specific managed care product offered by a payer
- Employer
- Patient's home ZIP code
- "Related" physicians

Case mix systems and cost accounting systems (discussed under criterion 7) usually are closely linked. Most cost accounting systems are able to perform case mix analyses, which enable health care organizations to examine costs associated with specific groupings of patient cases. An organization that has a case mix system, however, does not necessarily have associated cost accounting data. When cost accounting data are available, a case mix system becomes a "software engine" that converts raw cost accounting data to useful decision-support information.

The most effective way to demonstrate the value of case mix systems is to review the information generated by these systems. Tables 5 through 7 show sample reports generated by case mix systems.

The reports in tables 5 and 6 are physician specific. Physician-specific analyses are an especially important use of case mix data because physicians typically have the greatest influence over the resources utilized in a particular case (for example, days of care, type and number of tests, and so forth). Table 5

Table 5. Profitability by Physician Specialty

Specialty (Number of Cases)	Days	Patient Payment	Total Expected Total Cost	Net Profit
Orthopedics (240)	504.0	$ 537,600	$ 467,712	$ 69,888
Average per case	2.1	2,240	1,949	291
Internal medicine (165)	413.0	250,800	240,768	10,032
Average per case	2.5	1,520	1,459	61
Family practice (141)	310.0	186,402	180,810	5,592
Average per case	2.2	1,322	1,282	40
General surgery (82)	377.0	276,504	248,854	27,650
Average per case	4.6	3,372	3,035	337
OB/GYN (79)	166.0	112,812	115,068	(2,256)
Average per case	2.1	1,428	1,457	(29)
Cardiology (68)	367.0	342,992	315,553	27,439
Average per case	5.4	5,044	4,640	404
Gastroenterology (55)	94.0	81,565	76,671	4,894
Average per case	1.7	1,483	1,394	89
Report totals (830)	2,231.0	$1,788,675	$1,645,436	$143,239
Average per case	2.7	$ 2,155	$ 1,982	$173

Note: Specialties listed have 50 or more inpatient cases in the given time period.

Table 6. Treatment Protocol for Dr. Smith, DRG 127 (Heart Failure & Shock)

Procedure	Per-Case Procedure Volume	Procedure Charge per Unit	Procedure Cost per Unit	Average Charge per Case	Average Cost per Case
Nursing 3 West					
Private room 3 West	4.22	$278.00	$332.15	$1,173.16	$1,401.67
Semiprivate room 3 West	1.78	264.50	324.53	470.81	577.66
Nursing 3 West total	6.00			$1,643.97	$1,979.33
Intensive Care Unit					
Telemetry initial	0.67	$60.00	$118.05	40.20	79.09
Telemetry daily	1.22	25.00	96.35	30.50	117.55
Intensive care unit total	1.89			$70.70	$196.64
Emergency Room					
Intermediate exam	0.78	$52.00	$58.61	40.56	45.72
Monitor	0.67	29.50	40.52	19.77	27.15
ER clinical visits OP	1.00	0.00	0.00	0.00	0.00
Emergency room total	2.45			$60.33	$72.87
Respiratory Therapy					
STAT	0.11	$10.28	$3.96	$ 1.13	$ 0.41
Oxygen therapy	88.56	3.92	2.91	347.16	257.71
Updraft nebulizer charge	1.67	5.00	3.08	8.35	5.14
Sputum suction	0.11	22.82	6.06	2.51	0.67
Inhaler treatment	1.78	9.63	3.85	17.14	6.85
ER admit	0.67	9.63	3.85	6.45	2.58
Oximetry reading	0.22	27.29	6.81	6.00	1.50
Blood gas	2.11	53.50	11.20	112.89	23.63
Respiratory therapy total	95.23			$501.63	$298.49

Note: Procedures listed are for selected departments only.

analyzes net profitability by physician specialty and reveals that cardiology is most profitable with a net profit of $404 per case. Table 6 shows procedure-level detail for Dr. Smith's (a cardiologist) average clinical treatment protocol for a particular DRG. Table 7 analyzes inpatient and outpatient utilization and profitability by managed care plan.

What Is Needed to Answer Yes?

To answer yes and score two points for this criterion, your organization should have a case mix system in place that is able to produce reports similar to those shown in tables 5 through 7. (If cost accounting data are unavailable, then the cost information shown in those tables would not be needed to meet this criterion.) The case mix system also should have both of the following characteristics:

Table 7. Profitability by Managed Care Plan

Managed Care Plan	Number of Inpatient Cases	Number of Outpatient Cases	Expected Payments	Variable Cost	Total Cost	Net Profit	Marginal Profit
Community PHO	488	3,904	$1,456,192	$ 946,525	$1,368,820	$ 87,372	$ 509,667
Good Health HMO	425	3,188	1,588,700	1,080,316	1,509,265	79,435	508,384
Red Triangle HMO	276	2,484	1,207,224	700,190	1,122,718	84,506	507,034
Regional Health Plan	224	2,150	816,196	448,908	750,900	65,296	367,288
Retired People HMO	165	1,023	450,120	310,583	432,115	18,005	139,537
Premium PPO	121	1,029	348,550	247,470	338,093	10,457	101,080
Report totals	1,699	13,778	$5,866,982	$3,733,992	$5,521,911	$345,071	$2,132,990

Note: Plans analyzed had 100 or more inpatient cases in a given time period.

- Management can generate case mix reports easily and in a timely fashion (within an hour).
- The underlying patient database has a high degree of accuracy and the appropriate level of detail. Because accuracy and appropriateness are subjective attributes, management should attempt to develop suitable units of measure for this characteristic (for example, "employer and managed care plan identification information is entered upon admission or outpatient registration and is accurate for 99 percent of the cases").

In addition, your organization's case mix system should have at least two of the following three capabilities if you are to answer yes for this criterion:

1. The system can report physician-specific data for *each* physician associated with a particular case, including the admitting physician, attending physician, primary surgeon, at least two consulting physicians, and the resident (if there is a teaching program at the hospital). In addition, the system can analyze utilization based on a referring physician, which enhances the hospital's ability to profile physician utilization.
2. Resource utilization and other case mix information can be analyzed *by day of stay* for inpatient cases.
3. The system can analyze outpatient cases at levels of detail comparable to those of inpatient case analyses.

What about Partial Credit?

If your organization cannot meet all of the preceding requirements but can generate case mix reports by DRG and by admitting physician at least quarterly, then you can score one point for this criterion. However, if a significant portion of a case mix system's underlying patient data (medical records and billing information) is inaccurate or incomplete, then no points should be scored for this criterion.

Where Are Most Organizations Today?

Almost all hospitals can score at least one point on this criterion because most hospitals have case mix analysis capabilities. Two major aspects of case mix analysis are usually "under development" and are constantly being enhanced in hospitals:

1. Case mix analysis of ambulatory and off-site services
2. Linkage of supplemental systems and information—including cost accounting, outcomes measurement, patient satisfaction, and severity of illness data—with case mix systems

Case mix systems have proved to be a valuable resource for hospitals that have implemented and used them. To enhance the effectiveness of case mix systems as decision-support tools, health care organizations must continuously improve the accuracy and integrity of the underlying raw data. In addition, ongoing education and information sharing between management and physicians must be an integral part of case mix system implementation. Finally, as with cost accounting systems, the biggest future challenge will be the development of case mix systems across multiple sites for the full continuum of services, including inpatient and outpatient services, home care, long-term care, physician office services, and other ambulatory care center services.

Criterion 9

Information Readiness	No	In Progress/ Needs Improvement	Yes
9. Flexible reporting is available (for example, special reports can be produced easily).	0	1	2

Why Is Flexible Reporting Important?

A flexible report writer allows a user to extract selected information from a database, perform arithmetic operations on those data, and create various reports based on those data. In addition, a flexible report writer is an invaluable tool for the diagnosis and exploration of variances within a contracting organization, especially if the organization's information system tracks episodes of care. The diagnostic and exploratory aspects of flexible reporting are discussed in the following subsections.

Flexible Report Writer as a Diagnostic Tool

The most important aspect of managing under capitation is determining whether variations from budgets reflect normal fluctuations in activities or a process out of control. A flexible report writer can be used to "peel the onion" to find the root cause(s) of such variations.

For example, if a cost variance is noted during routine monthly monitoring of activity, a report can be designed to reveal what caused the variance. If frequency of service (for example, number of office visits per patient) appears to be a problem, the report writer can extract database information to reveal whether the problem's cause is *behavioral* (that is, based on differences in physician practice patterns) or *contractual* (that is, based on differences in benefits design among contracts with the same payer). If the problem is contractual, further diagnosis can reveal whether the problem relates to a specific contract (such as a contract with first-dollar coverage on physician office visits).

Once the cause of the variance is diagnosed, specific corrective actions can be implemented. Further, when an understandable, well-designed data report is shared with those who control the variation, the likelihood that corrective actions will be successful is enhanced greatly.

Another critical aspect of the diagnostic process is that data must be available as quickly as possible to catch problems before they become serious. Therefore, the diagnostic process should be part of a contracting organization's routine monthly financial reporting activity.

Flexible Report Writer as an Exploratory Tool

If a contracting organization accepts risk, its members must understand the economics of their organization as a whole in order to realize success. A flexible report writer enables an organization to gather and analyze data to develop such an understanding. For example, data can be analyzed to reveal possible weaknesses in the delivery of care, including variations in physician practice patterns, variations in consumption of health care resources, and redundant activities. Such data can serve as the basis for developing clinical guidelines to make the contracting organization more efficient and cost-effective. In addition, a flexible report writer allows the contracting organization to generate the credible, relevant information that can induce health care providers to change their behavior in order to ensure success under capitation.

What Is Needed to Answer Yes?

If your organization's information system has a report writer that is user-friendly (that is, it allows users to create reports on-line and is easy to use) and managers throughout your organization (including physicians) routinely access data through the report writer, answer yes and score two points for this criterion.

What about Partial Credit?

If your organization's information system has a flexible report writer but access to it is limited or if your organization currently is installing an information system with a flexible report writer, score one point for this criterion.

Criterion 10

Information Readiness	No	In Progress/ Needs Improvement	Yes
10. Hospital/system has a market database that provides profiles of area managed care plans, analyses of service area population and managed care enrollment, and competitor information.	0	1	2

Why Is Market Information Important?

A market database can help hospital management prepare for and compete in a capitated environment. Three major categories of information should be included in the development of any market database: profile of area managed care plans, distribution of the population by payer, and competitor utilization and financial information.

Hospitals need managed care plan information to truly understand the managed care players in the market and to know which plans currently capitate providers. This payer information enables a hospital to assess the magnitude of the risks associated with shifts in volume that may occur as plans convert to capitation or if exclusive contracts are developed and the hospital is excluded from a network.

A service area population profile is important to hospitals because market-share analysis under capitation focuses on the percentage of covered lives with which a hospital contracts, not the portion of total hospital admissions. Knowing area population distribution by payer should help hospital management answer the following questions:

- How many of a given HMO's enrolled lives are in our hospital's service area?
- Where exactly are the enrolled lives located?
- What is the age and sex distribution of the enrolled lives?

Five-year population profile forecasts also should be developed. Such forecasts need to highlight projected population increases; expected changes in managed care enrollment by plan; and anticipated conversions to managed care and capitation by Medicare, Medicaid, and major area commercial insurers.

A service area population profile, combined with information on area managed care plans and a hospital's internal data, enables an organization to develop an accurate estimate of its managed care and capitated market share. In addition, the population profile can facilitate the assessment of the strength of a health care system's geographic distribution of services relative to area payers' enrollees. The population profile and forecasts also should serve as the basis for a health care organization's development of economic models and financial forecasts.

The competitive financial and market-share data that most hospitals currently collect and evaluate become more important under capitation. Because profitability under capitation is achieved through cost management, understanding competitors' cost structures is critical to assessing competitors' likely success under capitation. The increased competition that typically accompanies a capitated environment requires hospitals to understand thoroughly the relative financial strengths and weaknesses of their competition.

What Is a Market Database?

A *market database* is any system that facilitates management's access to critical and timely market data. Data can be stored electronically in a computer database or manually in a filing cabinet. The following list outlines the basic data elements (grouped by the three categories of information previously mentioned) that should be included in an effective market database:

1. Profile of area managed care plans:
   - Name and location of managed care plan and contact names and phone numbers
   - Types and names of specific products offered (for example, HMO, POS)
   - Estimated total plan enrollment and, if possible, profile of enrollees (for example, employer, age and sex distribution, ZIP code of residence, and so forth)
   - Providers with whom the plan contracts and the providers' estimated share of enrollees
   - Payer's approach to physicians (for example, pricing, use of gatekeepers, employment of primary care providers, contracts with IPAs, and so forth)
   - Plan's hospital-specific historical utilization and pricing information
   - Plan's historical medical loss ratios
2. Distribution of population by payer:
   - Estimated distribution of current service area population by age/sex cohort and by payer and managed care plan
   - Forecast changes in population and payer/managed care enrollment
3. Competitor utilization and financial information:
   - Income statements, balance sheets, and financial ratios
   - Average charge per case by DRG
   - Productivity indicators
   - Inpatient and outpatient utilization trends and market share
   - Managed care activity

What Is Needed to Answer Yes?

To answer yes and score two points for this criterion, your hospital must have the data elements described in the preceding list in a current planning document or have the ability to produce such a report within minutes. In addition, *all* of the following requirements must be met:

1. The data within each of the market database's three major information categories reflect the most recent information available, and regular updates are performed.
2. An individual has been designated to be responsible for developing and maintaining the database.
3. Hospital management is aggressive and proactive in updating information on managed care plans and uses the following initiatives to review and update payer information: regularly scheduled meetings with the payers, a periodic written survey instrument, and telephone interviews.
4. Competitors' relative financial positions have been summarized, and competitor rankings have been established.
5. Summary market analyses are provided to board members and physicians on a regular basis.

What about Partial Credit?

The preceding five characteristics often represent the difference between simply having market data and using market information routinely and effectively. If your organization has market data available but the preceding five conditions are not met, then partial credit of one point should be scored. If significant effort is required to collect and/or organize raw market data, then no points should be scored.

Where Are Most Organizations Today?

Most hospitals that are active in managed care have at least a rudimentary database of area managed care plan information. Hospitals with excellent information tend to have good personal relationships with payers and are proactive and aggressive in obtaining market intelligence.

The availability of payer-specific information for small populations and geographic areas is limited. However, national data sources (for example, Interstudy) can be used as an excellent starting point in profiling area managed care providers. Local and regional business journals often provide detailed managed care estimates that are relevant to the local market. In addition, the state insurance commissioner's office usually has enrollment, premium, and medical loss ratio data. Further detail will require ongoing analysis and investigation by hospital management. Only a minority of hospitals have begun to analyze adequately their service area population at the payer and managed care plan level.

Competitor financial statements and comparative pricing (that is, charges) information are available in most markets. However, data on actual managed care payments to competitors usually are extremely difficult to obtain. The availability of market-share data and pricing information varies significantly by state, and comparative outpatient information is available in only a few states.

Related Issues

It is difficult for a hospital to obtain good information on area managed care plans, and it is especially difficult to obtain information on payers with whom the hospital does not currently contract. Personal relationships and politics play an important role in the development of a market database. A hospital's ultimate success in developing a strong database will depend in part on management's ability to identify the "right" individual to be responsible for obtaining market information.

Data on population distribution by payer will evolve over several years into a complete population-based database in which health-related information is maintained for each member of a hospital's service area population. This database will be linked eventually to the community health information networks envisioned for many markets.

Many financial managers have argued that comparative charge information is useless and that only cost comparisons are of value when assessing a hospital's relative competitive position for managed care and capitated contracts. Although the superior value of competitor cost data is unquestionable, these data rarely are available. Gross charges reflect relative resource consumption among specific case types within a hospital; therefore, comparisons based on charge data can be valid and useful in assessing a hospital's competitive position.

The usefulness of market databases will continue to improve as their accuracy and complexity increase. The key to developing an effective market database is to start now with whatever data are available and aggressively pursue enhanced information on an ongoing basis.

References and Notes

1. First Annual Aspen Symposium on Integrated Health Care. Aspen, Colorado, Mar. 29–30, 1993, quoted in The Advisory Board, *The Grand Alliance: Vertical Integration Strategies for Physicians and Health Systems,* Washington, DC: The Advisory Board Company, p. 23, 1993.

2. National Center for Health Statistics. *Advance Data, 1993 Summary. National Hospital Discharge Survey.* Hyattsville, MD: National Center for Health Statistics, May 24, 1995, p. 2.

3. Marion Merrill Dow. *Managed Care Digest/HMO Edition.* Kansas City, MO: Marion Merrill Dow, 1994, pp. 24–25.

4. Based on actual experience and targets of aggressive capitated systems in California, as reported by the Advisory Board Governance Committee.

5. The Advisory Board. *Capitation Strategy, Grand Alliance II.* Washington, DC: The Advisory Board Company, 1994, p. 114.

6. The Advisory Board, p. 115.

7. Burns, L. R., and Thorpe, D. P. Trends and models in physician–hospital organizations. *Health Care Management Review* 18(4):7–20, Fall 1993.

8. Covey, S. R. *The Seven Habits of Highly Effective People.* New York City: Fireside, 1989.

9. Axene, D. V., and Doyle, R. L. *Analysis of Medically Unnecessary Inpatient Services.* Seattle: Milliman & Robertson, 1994, p. 5.

10. Kostreski, F. Lowering C-section rates. collaboration the key. *AHA News* 30(24):7, June 13, 1994.

11. Davidson, J. Research mystery: use of surgery, hospitals varies greatly by region. *Wall Street Journal,* Mar. 5, 1986, sec. 2, p. 1.

12. Hudson, T. Growing pains. *Hospitals & Health Networks* 69(1):42–45, Jan. 5, 1995.

13. Paul Henchey, telephone interview with author, Amherst, MA, Oct. 1995.

14. Paul Henchey.

15. Information systems: the linchpin to prepaid success. *Capitation Management Report* 2(10):149–53, Oct. 1995.

16. Young, D. W., and Pearlman, L. K. Managing the stages of hospital cost accounting. *Healthcare Financial Management* 47(4):58, 60, 63–64, Apr. 1993.

17. Miller, T. R., and Ryan, J. B. Analyzing cost variance in capitated contracts. *Healthcare Financial Management* 49(2):22–23, Feb. 1995.

Suggested Readings

The Advisory Board. *Capitation Strategy, Grand Alliance II.* Washington, DC: The Advisory Board Company, 1994.

The Advisory Board. *Next Generation of Outcomes Tracking: Implications for Health Plans and Systems.* Washington, DC: The Advisory Board Company, 1994.

The Advisory Board. *Towards a Twenty-First Century Hospital: Redesigning Patient Care.* Washington, DC: The Advisory Board Company, Sept. 1992.

Agency for Health Care Policy and Research. *Agency for Health Care Policy and Research Guidelines.* Washington, DC: U.S. Government Printing Office, 1993–95.

Axene, D. V., and Doyle, R. L. *Analysis of Medically Unnecessary Inpatient Services.* Seattle: Milliman & Robertson, 1994.

Burns, L. R., and Thorpe, D. P. Trends and models in physician–hospital organizations. *Health Care Management Review* 18(4):7–20, Fall 1993.

Carpenter, C. E., and others. Cost accounting supports clinical evaluations. *Healthcare Financial Management* 48(4):40–44, Apr. 1994.

Clark, C. S. Planning along the continuum of care. *Healthcare Financial Management,* Aug. 1995, pp. 20–24.

Conklin, M. Health systems trying to fulfill data needs look to Sachs Group, Inforum. *Health Care Strategic Management* 12(6):9–10, June 1994.

Covey, S. R. *The Seven Habits of Highly Effective People.* New York City: Simon & Schuster, 1989.

Finkler, S. *Essentials of Cost Accounting for Health Care Organizations.* Gaithersburg, MD: Apsen, 1994.

Finkler, S. *Issues in Cost Accounting for Health Care Organizations.* Gaithersburg, MD: Aspen, 1994.

Goldberg, J. H. The new low-back guideline: the best you'll get? *Medical Economics* 72(15):161–70, Aug. 7, 1995.

Gottlieb, J. *Healthcare Cost Accounting Practice and Applications.* Westchester, IL: Healthcare Financial Management Association, 1989.

Government Accounting Office. *Hospital Costs: Cost Control Efforts at 17 Texas Hospitals.* Washington, DC: GAO, Dec. 1994.

Hastings, M. R. *Cost Management Strategies for Smaller Hospitals.* Chicago: American Hospital Publishing, 1993.

Hudson, T. Growing pains. *Hospitals & Health Networks,* Jan. 5, 1995.

Jennings Ryan & Kolb, Inc. (Peter F. Straley, ed.) *Developing a Successful Physician–Hospital Organization.* Chicago: American Hospital Publishing, 1995.

Marion Merrill Dow. *Managed Care Digest/HMO Edition.* Kansas City, MO: Marion Merrill Dow, 1994.

Milliman and Robertson, Inc. *M&R Healthcare Management Guidelines.* Vol. 1. *Inpatient and Surgical Care.* Milliman & Robertson, Sept. 1995.

Milliman and Robertson, Inc. *M&R Healthcare Management Guidelines.* Vol. 2. *Return-to-Work Planning.* Milliman & Robertson, Apr. 1994.

Milliman and Robertson, Inc. *M&R Healthcare Management Guidelines.* Vol. 3. *Ambulatory Care Guidelines.* Milliman & Robertson, Jan. 1994.

Milliman and Robertson, Inc. *M&R Healthcare Management Guidelines.* Vol. 4. *Home Care and Case Management.* Milliman & Robertson, June 1994.

National Committee for Quality Assurance. *Annual Member Health Care Survey Manual, Version 1.0.* Washington, DC: NCQA, 1995.

Tierney, W. M., and others. Predicting inpatient costs with admitting clinical data. *Medical Care,* Jan. 1995, pp. 1–14.

Tracking the System: American Health Care 1995. Washington, DC: National Committee for Quality Health Care, 1995.

Young, D. W., and Pearlman, L. K. Managing the stages of hospital cost accounting. *Healthcare Financial Management* 47(4):58, 60, 63–64, Apr. 1993.

About the Authors

Jennings Ryan & Kolb, Inc., is a management consulting firm providing services exclusively to the health care industry. The firm serves a national client base from offices in Atlanta; Chicago; Hadley, Massachusetts; and Jacksonville, Florida. Since Jennings Ryan & Kolb's inception in 1985, the firm has assisted hundreds of organizations along the continuum of health care, from acute care and specialty hospitals, to home health care companies and physician groups, to long-term care facilities. In the increasingly complex health care environment, Jennings Ryan & Kolb guides organizations toward integration of health care service delivery and financing. The firm has shared its expertise by providing faculty members for over 650 educational seminars and authoring over 80 articles and books, including *Developing a Successful Physician–Hospital Organization* (Chicago: American Hospital Publishing, 1995).

Marian C. Jennings is president of Jennings Ryan & Kolb. In her 17 years of consulting, Ms. Jennings has directed numerous strategic and financial planning initiatives for health care organizations across the United States. In addition, she is an expert in integrated delivery system development. Ms. Jennings has an MBA from Harvard University.

Deborah S. Kolb, PhD, is executive vice-president of Jennings Ryan & Kolb and executive-in-charge of the firm's Atlanta office. With over 16 years of health care consulting experience, Dr. Kolb has directed numerous strategic, financial, and integration planning projects. She frequently serves as faculty for seminars on topics such as affiliations and mergers, capitation and risk sharing, and health care industry trends. Dr. Kolb has an MBA and a PhD in English from the University of North Carolina at Chapel Hill.

J. Bruce Ryan is executive vice-president and cofounder of Jennings Ryan & Kolb. Mr. Ryan has over 19 years of health care management experience and is an expert in the areas of health care finance, capital management, valuation analysis, and strategic planning for managed care organizations. He is a frequent speaker on a wide variety of health care management topics including transitioning to capitation and capitation pricing. Mr. Ryan has a master of science degree in finance from the University of Massachusetts, Amherst, and a master of arts degree in economics from the University of Washington, Seattle.

Susanna E. Krentz is vice-president and executive-in-charge of Jennings Ryan & Kolb's Chicago office. Ms. Krentz has consulted extensively on strategy development and market positioning for hospitals and the formulation of managed care and integration strategies. She has an MBA from the University of Chicago.

Judith L. Horowitz is vice-president in the Atlanta office of Jennings Ryan & Kolb. Ms. Horowitz has over 13 years of health care management consulting experience and has consulted on a wide range of strategic, managed care, and integrated delivery system issues. She has an MBA from Vanderbilt University and an MA from the George Peabody College for Teachers, Nashville.

Margo P. Kelly is vice-president in the Jacksonville, Florida, office of Jennings Ryan & Kolb. Ms. Kelly has 11 years' experience consulting in the health care industry. Her consulting engagements have included program planning and financial analysis for a myriad of health care organizations and services. Prior to joining Jennings Ryan & Kolb, Ms. Kelly held administrative positions in both nonprofit and for-profit hospitals. She has an MBA and MHA from Tulane University.

Thomas R. Miller is a vice-president in Jennings Ryan & Kolb's Chicago office. He has consulted to a wide variety of health care organizations on issues including affiliations and mergers, managed care and strategic planning, and financial feasibility studies. Mr. Miller's prior experience includes serving as director of operations analysis for a proprietary hospital system and manager of decision support systems for a major health care consulting and computer firm. He has an MBA from the University of Rochester.

Cathy Sullivan Clark is vice-president and executive-in-charge of Jennings Ryan & Kolb's Hadley, Massachusetts, office. In her nine years as a management consultant, she has consulted on managed care issues to a wide range of provider organizations. Ms. Clark has a master of management degree from Northwestern University.

Heather L. Davidson is a consultant in the Atlanta office of Jennings Ryan & Kolb. She has participated in numerous hospital strategic planning projects including physician–hospital integration efforts. Ms. Davidson has an MBA and MHA from Georgia State University, Atlanta.

Scott B. Clay is a consultant in the Atlanta office of Jennings Ryan & Kolb. Mr. Clay has participated in a variety of strategic planning, affiliation, and managed care engagements. He has an MBA from Emory University.

Acknowledgments

Jennings Ryan & Kolb would like to acknowledge the many health care organizations with which it has had the pleasure to work. Its clients' confidence in the firm's ability to help them solve complex problems is what motivates and energizes the authors and the rest of the Jennings Ryan & Kolb staff.

This book reflects the experiences and efforts of many individual consultants within the firm. In addition, Erin Carr, research associate, assisted in verifying information and references. Finally, the authors would like to recognize the contribution of the firm's support staff, in particular, Michelle Middleton, who assisted in the production of the final manuscript, molding the parts into a smoother whole.